OXFORD MEDICAL PUBLIC~~~

The Management of Acute Pain

Second edition

GILBERT PARK
Department of Anaesthesia, Addenbrooke's Hospital, Cambridge

BARBARA FULTON
Department of Anaesthesia and Intensive Care, Newcastle General Hospital, Newcastle

and

SIVA SENTHURAN
Department of Anaesthesia, Addenbrooke's Hospital, Cambridge

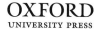

OXFORD
UNIVERSITY PRESS

OXFORD
UNIVERSITY PRESS

Oxford University Press
Great Clarendon Street, Oxford OX2 6DP
Oxford University Press is a department of the University of Oxford.
It furthers the University's objective of excellence in research, scholarship,
and education by publishing worldwide in
Oxford New York

Athens Auckland Bangkok Bogotá Buenos Aires Calcutta
Cape Town Chennai Dar es Salaam Delhi Florence Hong Kong Istanbul
Karachi Kuala Lumpur Madrid Melbourne Mexico City Mumbai
Nairobi Paris São Paulo Singapore Taipei Tokyo Toronto Warsaw
with associated companies in
Berlin Ibadan

Oxford is a registered trade mark of Oxford University Press
in the UK and in certain other countries

Published in the United States
by Oxford University Press, Inc., New York

© G. Park, B. Fulton, and S. Senthuran, 2000

The moral rights of the author have been asserted

Database right Oxford University Press (maker)

First edition published 1991
Second edition published 2000

British Library Cataloguing in Publication Data
Data available

Library of Congress Cataloging in Publication Data
Park, G. R. (Gilbert R.)
The management of acute pain/Gilbert Park, Barbara Fulton,
and Siva Senthuran.—2nd ed.
p. ; cm.—(Oxford medical publications)
Includes bibliographical references and index.
1. Analgesics. 2. Pain—Chemotherapy. 3. Analgesia. I. Fulton, Barbara.
II. Senthuran, Siva. III. Title. IV. Series.
[DNLM: 1. Pain—drug therapy. 2. Analgesics—therapeutic use. 3. Anesthesia,
Local—methods. 4. Anesthetics, Local—therapeutic use. WL 704 P235m 2000]
RM319.P37 2000   616'.0472—dc21   00-032694

1 3 5 7 9 10 8 6 4 2

ISBN 0 19 262467 9 (Pbk)

Typeset by
Phoenix Photosetting, Chatham, Kent

Printed in Great Britain on acid free paper by
T. J. International Ltd, Padstow

616.0472
p

TO5599

Preface to the second edition

Since the first edition, acute pain control has improved. For this second edition we therefore recruited the help of others including Dr S. Bass, Dr R. Munglani, and specialist nurses, R. Sapsford and S. Kinna. Also, one of us (B.F.) has moved to Newcastle. Thus we decided to broaden the outlook of the book whilst keeping the style of this edition the same as the first. Dr Anne Coleman has added a chapter on the acute pain service.

There are more illustrations and we are grateful to Mr P. Ball for his drawings. Finally, we thank those reviewers in the various journals who took the time and trouble to read our first edition. We have taken on board some, but not all, of their criticisms.

In addition to these changes, we have rewritten extensive parts of the book and reordered some chapters to make the text flow easier and more in keeping with clinical practice.

Cambridge and Newcastle   S.S.
2000   B.F.
                                                            G.R.P.

Preface to the first edition

The aim of this book is to provide simple practical guidance for those who prescribe and administer drugs for acute pain relief, particularly junior medical and nursing staff. This book is not intended as a comprehensive review of the subject or to replace current texts, but as a practical problem-orientated guide to an important subject, which is often poorly understood and inadequately managed. Within the limits of this book's size, it is impossible to include every problem that may arise, but the information contained we hope provides a logical approach to any acute pain problem.

Drug dosages have been included for many drugs. Despite careful checking, mistakes may have occurred and if a dose appears incorrect it should be checked with the package insert, British National Formulary, or other suitable reference source, before the drug is administered.

We gratefully acknowledge the assistance and co-operation of the many medical and nursing staff, especially Mr P. Doyle, Dr M.J. Lindop, and Sisters D. Pick and S. Bothamley, from whom we have received many helpful suggestions during the preparation of this book.

Cambridge   B.F.
1991   G.R.P.

Contents

1

Why is pain control a problem?

Numerous studies of hospital patients have confirmed that acute pain is often inadequately managed. Patients of all ages experience considerable pain during their hospital admissions, despite the widespread availability of drugs and techniques to relieve pain. The reasons for ineffective pain control in hospitals have been a source of much speculation and study. Some of the major reasons which have been considered follow.

Lack of knowledge or interest in pain control

- Lack of understanding of the nature and pathophysiology of pain and methods of control.
- Lack of knowledge of the pharmacology of analgesic drugs and of alternative methods of administration available to improve drug efficacy can lead to inadequate prescriptions and poor analgesia.
- Lack of practical skill, not allowing regional analgesic techniques to be used.
- Lack of knowledge of adjuvant techniques and drugs to improve pain control.

Failure to assess pain relief accurately

The provision of analgesia is often dependent upon assessment by a third party, nurse, or doctor. Judgements about the severity of pain may be made with no reference to the individual patient. One condition may be considered to be less painful than another and therefore less analgesia will be prescribed or administered. There is often no review of the adequacy of pain control or the effectiveness of analgesic drug regimes. Prescriptions may be written but then there may be little follow-up of the effect on the individual patient.

Failure of communication

Patients must communicate their need for analgesia to the staff who are responsible for their care. There may be a number of reasons for a patient failing to do this including not wanting to be seen to complain, the belief that it may be cowardly to need analgesia, or a simple lack of understanding of how to obtain analgesia. The ward staff also have a responsibility to communicate the facilities available for analgesia and how the patient may obtain help. Both sides may fail to communicate with each other.

Fear of addiction to analgesics

Fear of addiction often leads medical and nursing staff to administer less analgesics to patients. Patients themselves may be concerned about this and consequently do not request sufficient drug to adequately control their pain. This fear frequently stems from a lack of knowledge of the true risks of addiction in patients who are receiving opioid drugs for the management of acute pain. Such addiction is extremely rare; it should not be used as an excuse for withholding opioid analgesics.

Fear of unwanted drug effects

The risks of unwanted effects such as respiratory depression with opioid drugs or gastrointestinal haemorrhage with non-steroidal anti-inflammatory drugs may often lead to inadequate drug administration.

Fear of masking physical signs

This problem may arise in a patient admitted as an emergency, where the fear of masking physical signs and making the diagnosis difficult is used as a reason for withholding analgesia. The patient with acute peritonitis may not be given analgesia 'until the surgeon has assessed him'. This is an unfounded fear. Analgesia does not mask physical signs.

The value of suffering

Some pain is expected as part of most illness or particularly after surgery and trauma. The goal of no pain is often seen as unachievable. Both patients and staff may have developed attitudes like 'pain is good for you!' that associate suffering with self improvement. This is clearly not so.

Legal aspects of drug administration

Procedures for the administration of controlled drugs may often be inhibiting to staff and patients. Shortage of staff to check the drugs and fear of disciplinary actions if records are incorrect may add to delays and concern over the administration of opioid analgesics. In addition, the patient appreciating the amount of work this means for nursing staff may refrain from asking for analgesia.

A PRACTICAL APPROACH TO PROBLEM PAIN

This section is designed to introduce guidelines to the nurse or doctor involved in the management of patients in pain. Individual chapters of this book will deal in more detail with drugs and techniques that are mentioned here.

After dealing with the cause of the pain to the best of one's ability, a suitable analgesic needs to be selected. The advantages and disadvantages of the different analgesic agents are listed in Table 1.1. and Fig. 1.1 shows the sites of action of these analgesic agents.

In selecting a suitable analgesic agent, the following have to be borne in mind.

Severity of pain: the pain control 'ladder'

The concept of the 'ladder' of pain control originated from the management of patients with chronic pain. However, it provides a useful guideline for acute pain (see Fig. 1.2).

Table 1.1 The main advantages and disadvantages of analgesic agents

Mode used	Main advantages	Main disadvantages
Paracetamol (Chapter 11)	Analgesic, antipyretic, very few side-effects, easily administered.	Weak analgesic. No anti-inflammatory properties.
Codeine (Chapter 7)	Weak opioid, respiratory depression rare.	Sedation, weak analgesic, constipation.
Non-steroidal anti-inflammatory drugs (Chapter 11)	Moderately potent analgesics and anti-inflammatory drugs. No respiratory depression. No sedation.	Gastric erosions and renal failure are serious side-effects. Not useful in all types of pain e.g. phantom limb pain.
Opioids (Chapter 7)	Very potent analgesics. Relieve most types of pain.	Respiratory depression, sedation, constipation, nausea, and vomiting are main side-effects. Abuse and addiction potential, so legal controls.
Local anaesthetics (Chapter 12)	No respiratory depression or sedative effects. Effectively block pain perception in a selected area only.	Needs skill and monitoring to be administered effectively as part of regional block. Risk of local anaesthetic toxicity with large doses or continuous infusions.

Mode used	Main advantages	Main disadvantages
Transcutaneous electrical nerve stimulation (TENS) (Chapter 18)	No adverse effects. Commonly used in labour.	Expensive equipment. No proof of analgesic efficacy.
Inhaled Entonox (Chapter 18)	Good analgesic for short-term procedural pain e.g. labour/dressing changes. Rapid onset and offset of analgesia.	Needs cylinder/pipeline supply. Patient co-operation needed. Euphoria and nausea.
Psychological techniques (Chapter 4)	No adverse effects.	Requires training and time of dedicated counsellor. Useful in select groups of patients only e.g. children and motivated adults.

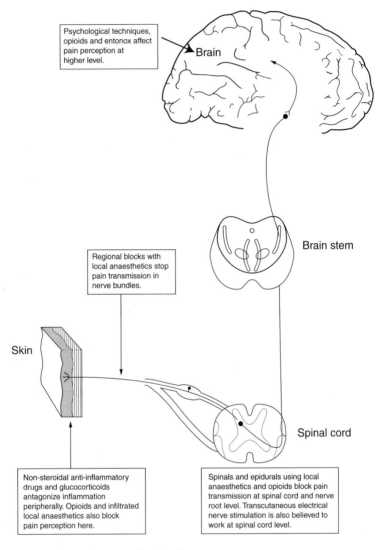

Psychological techniques, opioids and entonox affect pain perception at higher level.

Brain

Regional blocks with local anaesthetics stop pain transmission in nerve bundles.

Brain stem

Skin

Non-steroidal anti-inflammatory drugs and glucocorticoids antagonize inflammation peripherally. Opioids and infiltrated local anaesthetics also block pain perception here.

Spinals and epidurals using local anaesthetics and opioids block pain transmission at spinal cord and nerve root level. Transcutaneous electrical nerve stimulation is also believed to work at spinal cord level.

Spinal cord

Fig. 1.1 Sites of action of analgesics.

Acute pain can be divided into mild, moderate, severe, and very severe. Any individual can be sited along this ladder of pain at any time. Patients with acute pain will tend to go down the ladder with time, as pain tends to decrease with time. This is unlike the patient

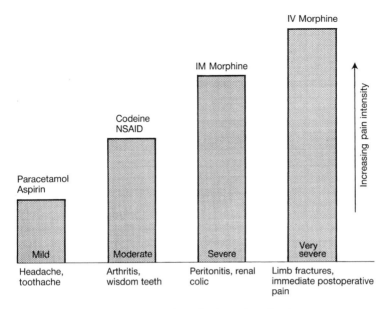

Fig. 1.2 A graphical representation of pain and analgesia.

with chronic pain from malignancy who may climb the ladder as increasingly potent analgesics are required to control the worsening pain associated with the progression of the disease.

At the bottom of the ladder is 'minor' pain typified by a headache or toothache. This would usually be well controlled by oral drugs, most commonly the non-steroidal anti-inflammatory agents such as aspirin or paracetamol. Climbing the ladder, with pain of increasing severity, more potent analgesic drugs will be required.

For moderate pain, oral drugs may still be sufficient and the oral opioids such as codeine may be used. In addition, the combination of oral opioids with aspirin and paracetamol is widely used. Codeine in combination with paracetamol has been shown to provide better analgesia than paracetamol alone. Such drugs would be helpful in the patient with pain following the extraction of wisdom teeth, for example.

Severe pain in the hospital setting is usually an indication for systemic administration of opioid drugs or where suitable, a regional anaesthetic block. Morphine is the standard opioid drug to which other agents are compared. Pain associated with trauma or postoperative pain is commonly managed by intermittent doses of intramuscular opioids. Very severe pain immediately after surgery, or in trauma patients after limb fractures, or breakthrough pain is best controlled by intravenous opioid analgesics to produce rapid improvement in analgesia or a regional analgesic technique.

Choice of route of administration

This depends on both the drug formulations and the resources for patient care that are available. In acute, severe pain the intravenous route should be used for the immediate control of pain once it has become established. Frequent intramuscular administration of analgesics gives effective analgesia and does not require the same technical skills and intravenous access. It may be a useful and practical method once the pain has been controlled with an intra- venous bolus. Epidural analgesia is also useful for severe pain after abdominal, pelvic, or lower limb surgery but requires staff trained to monitor patients for dangerous complications like respiratory depression and hypotension. Oral and rectal administration are more appropriate routes for providing prolonged analgesia in ambulant patients.

Treat the patient, not the symptom

Each patient is an individual. Pain control must be tailored to his or her requirements. This begins with a careful, complete evaluation of the patient, and requires frequent assessment of the patient's response to pain and its improvement with analgesics.

Pain should be treated according to what the patient feels and not what their attendants think they should feel.

Allow for individual variability

Drug response may differ widely between patients. The reasons for this are complex and poorly understood. The patient's response to an analgesic may also vary according to the illness. Age-related changes have been documented and generally older patients require less frequent analgesia than young patients. Standard prescriptions of analgesic drugs are therefore unhelpful and drug administration must be modified to suit the individual patient.

Be aware of the pharmacology of drugs

It is important to have a knowledge of basic drug pharmacology. Factors such as the time of onset of drug action and the duration of analgesic effect are important considerations when prescribing analgesic drugs. How do the agents produce their analgesic effect? What are the unwanted effects associated with their use? All of these factors must be considered when prescribing analgesics.

Useful drug combinations

Opioid drugs administered in combination with non-steroidal anti-inflammatory drugs, antihistamines, or tricyclic antidepressant drugs can improve analgesic efficacy.

Administer analgesic drugs regularly

Infrequent, intermittent administration of analgesic drugs will result in intervals of pain between doses. If this is combined with an 'on demand' prescription, the patient must wait until pain is experienced before asking for further analgesia. Frequent, regular doses of analgesic will go a considerable way towards improving pain control.

Use of local analgesic techniques

Useful techniques for providing analgesia using local anaesthetic agents are discussed in Chapter 13. The assistance of personnel skilled in the more complex techniques, such as thoracic epidural analgesia, may usually be sought from the department of anaesthesia, the intensive care unit, or from the pain control clinics that are becoming widely established in most hospitals.

Non-pharmacological techniques

Adjuvant psychological techniques such as relaxation and hypnosis may be appropriate in difficult patients. Assistance from interested and appropriately trained personnel will be required.

Careful monitoring and management of unwanted effects

This is mandatory whatever means are employed to treat acute pain. Staff involved in patient care must be well practised in resuscitation and in the recognition and treatment of the specific problems relating to drugs and techniques used to provide analgesia.

2
What is pain?

DEFINITION OF PAIN

Pain is felt by all human beings on occasions. Usually it is of a minor nature (such as a headache or muscle strain) and improves quickly without pharmacological intervention. Rarely it is severe, usually following injury or after a surgical operation, and intensive pharmacological efforts may be needed to relieve the pain and distress. Thus we are all familiar with what pain is.

In scientific terms pain has been defined by the International Association for the Study of Pain (IASP) as 'an unpleasant sensory and emotional experience associated with actual or potential tissue damage, or described in terms of such damage'.

A painful stimulus is a protective response for the individual. Those with diminished or altered pain sensitivity may sustain severe joint injury and deformity or other tissue damage like burns because of the lack of pain sensation.

PHYSIOLOGY AND NEUROPHARMACOLOGY OF PAIN

Several factors must be considered when the topic of how pain is evoked and perceived is discussed. The interaction of the following is important:

- The peripheral pain sensors (nociceptors).
- Pain-producing (algesic) substances.
- Sensitization of nerve endings.

- The pathway taken by pain impulses to the sensory cortex of the brain.
- Neurotransmitters

The peripheral pain sensors

The two main types of nociceptors are mechanoreceptors and polymodal nociceptors.

Mechanoreceptors are mainly present in the skin and respond to strong pressure applied to a wide area of skin and strong stimuli such as a pinprick and sudden application of heat (greater than 44°C). They warn of potential damage and are the afferent part of the withdrawal reflexes. This type of receptor is associated with small myelinated primary afferent neurones designated Aδ (delta) type. These neurones transmit impulses rapidly. Stimulation of this type of receptor results in 'first' or 'rapid' pain which occurs almost immediately after injury and is usually sharp, localized, and pricking.

Polymodal nociceptors are the nerve endings of unmyelinated primary afferent neurones of the C type. They are widely distributed throughout most tissues and the classification as polymodal indicates that they respond to tissue damage caused by mechanical, thermal, or chemical insults. In addition, they respond to chemical mediators formed or released as a result of tissue damage. These impulses are transmitted more slowly than impulses from the mechanoreceptors and travel along unmyelinated C-type nerve fibres. It is these impulses, from polymodal nociceptors, which are responsible for 'second' or 'slow' pain that is slower in onset, prolonged, dull, aching poorly localized and occurs after injury.

Pain-producing (algesic) substances

Algesic substances are released by damaged tissues and either directly or indirectly evoke pain. They include substances such as bradykinin, acetylcholine, and potassium ions (which can directly stimulate the sensory nerve endings) as well as prostaglandins (which can potentiate the effect of stimuli but do not directly cause pain themselves). Others, like substance P, can increase the permeability of local blood vessels and produce local extravasation.

Sensitization of nerve endings

When an injury is inflicted, pain is first evoked by the stimulation of the nociceptors as well as the release of algesic substances in a localized area. This phenomenon is known as primary hyper-algesia. As healing starts, nerve endings of the polymodal C fibres show increased sensitivity to stimuli. Thus any stimulus in a wider area than the initial site of injury becomes painful. This process is a result of increased sensitization of nerve endings and is known as secondary hyperalgesia.

Pain pathways

Pain impulses are mainly carried by Aδ and C fibres which enter the spinal cord through the dorsal root where their cell bodies are located. After entering the spinal cord most of the Aδ and C fibres terminate superficially by synapsing with other neurones in the grey matter of the dorsal horn. The majority of both Aδ and C fibres synapse either directly or, more frequently, via intermediate neurones in the deeper layers of the dorsal horn, with ascending fibres which cross the midline to join the spinothalamic and spino-reticular tracts (Fig. 2.1).

The spinal cord is not just a relay station for impulses, but is also involved in the processing of impulses (like the brain). Complex circuits consisting of neurones synapsing with other neurones exist in the dorsal horn. The details of synapses and connections in the dorsal horn are complex and beyond the scope of this book.

Pain transmission can be inhibited at the spinal cord level by inhibitory interneurones that lie within the spinal cord or from descending inhibitory fibres originating from the brain. The best known theory describing how painful stimuli may be altered at the spinal level is the 'gate theory' put forward by Melzack and Wall in 1965. They postulated that painful stimuli have to pass through a 'gate' in order to be relayed on to the central nervous system (see Fig. 2.2) This gate can be closed by non-painful sensory input carried by large myelinated fibres (Aβ fibres) from mechano-receptors responding to low-threshold stimuli such as the immediate tactile response of 'rubbing it better'.

This is how transcutaneous electrical nerve stimulators (TENS) are thought to work. In TENS the mechanoreceptors in the nerve

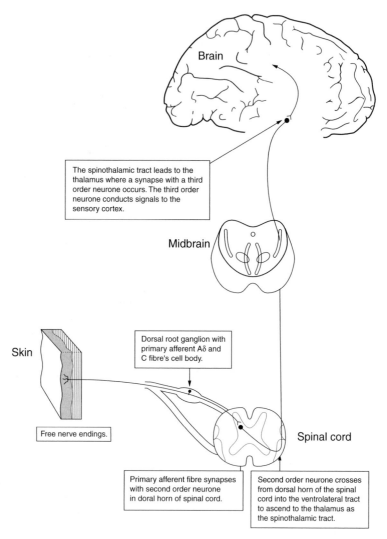

Fig. 2.1 Simplified pain transmission pathway (the oligosynaptic pathway).

distribution of a painful stimulus (for instance, a surgical incision) are stimulated by a low-intensity electrical stimulation with the result that the gate is closed to the passage of the painful stimuli. In addition, the gate may be closed as a result of descending inhibitory systems that originate in the brain.

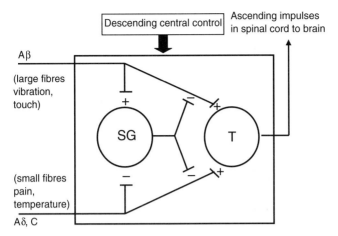

Fig. 2.2 A Gate control theory of pain: nerve impulses transmitted by the small fibres (Aδ, C) inhibit the substantia gelatinosa (SG) cell and stimulate the first central transmission cell (T), thereby opening the gate to the brain. Impulses in the large fibres (Aβ), stimulate the T cell and the inhibitory SG cell. The SG cell then releases inhibitory neurotransmitters at its endings, decreasing the stimulation of the T cell by small and large fibre impulses, thereby closing the gate. Thus the balance of large fibre input, small fibre input, and descending central control from the brain (e.g. emotion, memory) influence the pain signals transmitted through the gate to the brain. Inhibitory (−) neurotransmitters hyperpolarize cells whereas excitatory (+) neurotransmitters depolarize cells.

Ascending pain impulses are transmitted mainly through the spinothalamic tract. Fibres from the dorsal horn project to lateral and medial areas of the thalamus from where further transmission of impulses is to areas of the sensory and motor cortex. This is the major route of sensory–discriminatory potential. Fibres that project in this way tend to be fast conducting, have few synapses, and belong to the oligosynaptic (or lemniscal) system of pain pathways.

Ascending impulses may also travel via the spinoreticular tract and they do so more slowly, terminating in the pontomedullary reticular formation. These impulses have a major role in the arousal/motivational aspects of pain sensation, resulting from their connections with the limbic system. They are also responsible for the autonomic effects associated with pain resulting from the responses of the hypothalamus. Fibres that project in this way tend to be slow conducting, have many intermediate synapses before they reach the sensory cortex, and belong to the multisynaptic (or non-lemniscal) system of pain pathways.

Descending pathways are mainly inhibitory in nature. Stimuli are produced in response to cortical and subcortical activation responding to sustained peripheral pain input. These descending impulses are visualized as 'gate' controls, thereby modulating pain input.

Neurotransmitters and pain

At the spinal cord level the principal neurotransmitter involved in the transmission of pain impulses is substance P. The excitatory amino acids, especially aspartate and glutamate, also play an important role in pain transmission. Other transmitters which have been identified include angiotensin II, somatostatin, cholecystokinin (CCK), enkephalins and dynorphins of the endogenous opioid peptides, 5-hydroxy tryptamine (5HT), and noradrenaline (norepinephrine).

The chemical modulation of nociceptive impulses is complex. The place of agonist and antagonist drugs related to the neurotransmitters in the control of pain transmission is still undergoing evaluation. The hope that chemical modifications of the endogenous opioid peptides may lead to the development of an analgesic agent with few side-effects remains the goal of many investigators in this area.

ENDOGENOUS OPIOID PEPTIDES AND THEIR RECEPTORS

The observation that exogenous compounds like morphine have analgesic activity at very low concentrations and that there are stereospecific molecules of morphine led to the search for opioid receptors. The discovery of opioid receptors then led to the search for the endogenous molecules that bind to these receptors.

At present three main opioid receptors have been identified. These have been classified as μ, δ, and κ. In an attempt to unify opioid receptor classification, the International Union of Pharmacology (IUPHAR) has reclassified opioid receptors as OP_1 (δ), OP_2 (κ), and OP_3 (μ). The main effects of the opioid receptors are shown in Table 2.1.

Table 2.1 The main effects of opioid receptor activation

Receptor *	Effects	Agonist	Antagonist
OP$_3$ (μ)	Supraspinal and peripheral analgesia Respiratory depression Constipation ↑ Gut secretions ↓ Baroreceptor reflexes	Morphine	Naloxone
OP$_1$ (δ)	Supraspinal and peripheral analgesia ? Respiratory stimulant Constipation ↓ Gut secretions ↓ Blood pressure	Leu-enkephalin	Naloxone
OP$_2$ (κ)	? Supraspinal analgesia ↑ Spinal pain transmission ↓ Intestinal peristalsis ↓ Intestinal secretions	Dynorphin Ketocyclazocine	Unknown

* Note that the σ receptor is no longer considered an opioid receptor.

About 20 endogenous opioid peptides that bind to these receptors have also been discovered. These are derived from three main families of peptides known as the pro-enkephalin family, the pro-opiomelanocortin family, and the pro-dynorphin family. The role of the endogenous opioid peptides is yet to be characterized fully. The endogenous opioid peptides appear to be mixed agonists with effects resulting from actions at more than one opioid receptor subtype. The main peptides from each of the families are:

Enkephalins
These are five-amino-acid peptides derived from the pro-enkephalin family. They have an extensive distribution in the CNS and are found spinally and supraspinally.

β Endorphin
This is a 31-amino-acid peptide derived from the pro-opiomelano-cortin family. This is an unusual opioid in that it has a limited distribution and is primarily restricted to a hypothalamic cell group.

Dynorphins

This is a third class of endogenous opioid peptides derived from the pro-dynorphin family. Their actions are mainly at spinal cord level.

Functions of the endogenous opioids

The opioid receptors and opioid peptides have been implicated in a number of homeostatic functions of the body including:

Analgesia

The role of endogenous opioid peptides in mediating analgesia is not clear. However, in the periphery (that is, in the tissues outside the brain and spinal cord) μ receptor activation by opioid drugs inhibits the sensitization of nociceptors by inflammatory mediators like prostaglandin E_2. In the spinal cord and in the brain, μ and δ receptors seem to mediate analgesia whereas κ receptor activation seems to potentiate pain transmission.

Respiration

The centres in the medulla controlling breathing have μ and δ receptors, activation of which causes respiratory depression. The κ receptor seems to have minimal involvement with the respiratory centre. Naloxone (which is an opioid receptor antagonist) given to neonates stimulates breathing suggesting that the endogenous opioid peptides may have a regulatory role in depressing the ventilatory drive.

Cardiovascular system

The role of the opioids in cardiovascular regulation is suggested by the observation that μ receptor activation attenuates the baro-receptor reflexes that maintain blood pressure. Naloxone also reverses the decrease in blood pressure during shock — though with no long-term benefit. Overall, opioid receptor activation seems to act as a depressor, especially when the sympathetic tone is high.

Gastrointestinal system

Activation of the μ and δ receptors in the brain and spinal cord by opioid drugs results in constipation. Activation of μ and κ receptors in the gastrointestinal tract decreases peristalsis of the gut and δ receptor activation results in decreased gastrointestinal tract secretions.

Endocrine system

Opioids have been found to decrease the secretion of adreno-corticotrophic hormone (ACTH) by the posterior pituitary gland as well as inhibit the release of antidiuretic hormone (ADH) by the anterior pituitary in response to increased blood osmolarity.

CLINICAL ASPECTS OF PAIN

Pain in some form will be treated by clinicians of almost every discipline. The varied causes of pain and the clinical settings with which it is associated may result in different perceptions of pain. As a consequence analgesic therapy may need to be adjusted accordingly.

Trauma

The assessment of pain in trauma victims shows that it varies greatly depending upon the cause. Often little pain may be felt at the time of injury, e.g. a soldier wounded in battle or a fireman injured during the rescue of a child from a burning building may feel little immediate pain. However, the innocent civilian involved in a train crash or a bomb blast will complain of considerably more pain and may also require sedation because of the psychological and emotional shock of the incident.

The explanation of this phenomenon may be partly psychological i.e. the need to get away from the cause of the injury overriding the pain and its immobilizing reflexes, and the need for involvement in the event for the soldier or fireman. In addition, pain and stress will also stimulate the release of endogenous opioids in the central nervous system, and these modify the pain response.

Early and effective analgesia is needed after trauma, preferably at the scene of the accident. Small (1–2 mg) boluses of morphine or other opioid should be given intravenously and titrated to analgesic effect while awaiting surgical treatment. The importance of immobilizing fractures as a means of controlling pain should not be forgotten. Modern surgical assessment is less dependent on clinical signs as radiological techniques are widely available to aid in diagnosis. Patients with a head injury and those suffering continuing blood loss should have even smaller boluses of morphine (0.5–1 mg) as loss of consciousness or hypotension can occur with analgesia. Titrating small doses of opioid is safer than administering large (e.g. 10 mg) standard doses. Furthermore, intravenous administration is safer and more reliable in trauma as absorption from subcutaneous and intramuscular sites can be impaired because of hypoperfusion.

Surgical pain

Adequate pain relief following surgery is essential for a rapid and uncomplicated recovery. The severity of postoperative pain is influenced by many factors which are listed below.

1. **Site of operation**. Abdominal and thoracic surgical procedures are considerably more painful than peripheral and body-surface surgery.
2. **Time of day of surgery**. Morning operations are associated with less discomfort than those performed in the afternoon. This may be a result of diurnal variation in the concentrations of steroid hormones or modifications in the stress response to surgery. These effects may be mediated through the endogenous opioid peptide system.
3. **Sex differences**. The majority of studies of acute pain have demonstrated that female patients report higher pain scores than male patients after equivalent operations. However, other studies have shown no difference in analgesic requirements between the sexes.
4. **Previous pain experience**. There is a general expectation of pain after surgery. However, if patients have been in considerable pain from their illness or injury, which is relieved by surgery, postoperative pain may be less. Some patients with a background of chronic pain may experience more pain than would be expected after an acute injury or after surgery.
5. **Character of the pain**. Colicky, intermittent pain is less easily tolerated than continuous pain.
6. **Individual psychological factors**. These are discussed in Chapter 4.

Emergency surgery

The factors mentioned above will also apply to the patient who has just had emergency surgery, but there may be additional factors, some of which are listed below.

- Greater fear and anxiety may be aroused by the nature of the emergency. For example, after road traffic accidents the fear of blame may be a considerable concern that increases the emotional distress associated with the pain.
- In some emergency situations the patient may have little or no time to worry, which may lessen the impact of pain.
- Patients who have multiple injuries may have depression of their conscious level which will decrease pain perception.

NON-TRAUMATIC PAIN

Patients with medical conditions unrelated to surgery or trauma may also suffer from acute pain and these illnesses similarly require appropriate analgesic therapy.

Myocardial infarction

The severe pain of myocardial infarction is an indication for opioid analgesia. Although modern research has concentrated upon methods of improving perfusion to the ischaemic myocardium with the use of intravenous thrombolytic agents and coronary angioplasty, the pain, distress, and anxiety that accompany the myocardial ischaemia will result in an increase in sympathetic tone and release of catecholamines. The accompanying tachycardia, dysrhythmias, hypertension, and increased myocardial work may worsen the ischaemia and hasten myocardial cell death. Thus the judicious use of opioid analgesics in these patients can improve cardiovascular function.

The central effects of analgesics, by reducing the response to pain, will decrease sympathetic tone and catecholamine production. This, in turn, will reduce the pre-load and after-load on the heart. When morphine is used the vasodilatation will further reduce myocardial work. However, in a few patients, analgesic agents may produce significant hypotension after myocardial infarction. The central mood-elevating effects of opioid drugs will also play an important role in alleviating anxiety in patients.

The good and bad effects of opioids in acute myocardial infarction can be summarized as:

Good effects

- Analgesia
- Anxiolysis
- Antiarrhythmic
- Vasodilator (decreases work of heart)

Bad effects

- Sedation
- Hypotension
- Nausea and vomiting

The choice of analgesic agent will depend upon the patient's level of pain, haemodynamic state, and respiratory stability, and how the drug may be expected to modify these parameters. Opioids are generally the standard agents and morphine and diamorphine the most widely used. These should be given intravenously; intramuscular administration may result in variable absorption and widespread bruising if the patient is receiving thrombolytic therapy.

Nausea and vomiting may counteract the benefits of the opioids, so an appropriate antiemetic should be administered with them (Chapter 19). Dysphoria may also be seen after the administration of some opioids and this may result in unwanted restlessness and agitation.

Inflammatory pain

Examples of acutely painful inflammatory conditions include acute pancreatitis and acute arthritis (rheumatoid, gout, etc.). The inflammatory process leads to the formation of tissue oedema which, with increasing tissue tension, results in pain. In addition, substances released during inflammation and cell damage, such as histamine, prostaglandins, substance P, 5-hydroxy tryptamine (5HT), and kinins make the afferent nerve endings more sensitive.

Opioid drugs may be needed to control severe pain from these causes. This type of pain may also benefit from non-steroidal anti-inflammatory drugs (NSAIDs) for both their analgesic and anti-inflammatory properties. Drugs such as indomethacin, diclofenac, piroxicam, and naproxen may be used in addition to opioids or on their own in less painful conditions. Acute gout is usually treated with high doses of NSAIDs.

Visceral pain

The differences in the transmission pathways of pain impulses from viscera result in pain of a different quality and character to that resulting from other forms of injury. Visceral pain impulses are transmitted in fibres that are predominantly unmyelinated and found in sympathetic nerves. These can impinge on somatic input from the relevant dermatomes at spinal cord level and from there project to the brain in both the spinoreticular and spinothalamic tracts. There may be discomfort (with or without pain) resulting from this, which is characteristically poorly localized.

THE ASSESSMENT OF PAIN

Pain is a sensation which is difficult to express and quantify. Further difficulties occur with its study since individual patients will have a different perception and emotional response to similar painful stimuli.

In some patients the cause of the pain will be immediately obvious (a trauma patient with a broken leg, for example); in others a complete history of the pain will be needed if it is to be adequately treated. The features that may be helpful in the diagnosis and assessment are shown in Table 2.2.

Once the pain has been characterized its severity can be evaluated using one of two approaches.

1. Subjective measurements

These rely mainly on the patients' expression of their pain. There are two basic methods available.

Descriptive scales

These vary greatly in complexity but essentially consist of a series of words describing pain severity from 'no pain' to 'severe'. One example of a simple scale suitable for clinical use would be:

1   No pain
2   Mild pain
3   Moderate pain
4   Severe pain

Table 2.2 Clinical features of pain used in diagnosis and assessment

Onset	Gradual, sudden.
Main site	Chest, abdomen, limbs, wound pain, etc.
Radiation	Pain may also appear to radiate to areas distant from the principal site. The pain of angina pectoris, for example, typically radiates to the neck, jaw, and arm; ureteric pain may radiate from the loin region into the groin; hip pain may also be felt in the region of the knee.
Character	Pain may vary in character and common descriptions include colicky, knife-like, constant, burning, etc.
Severity	Pain severity may be evaluated from the patient's descriptive terms — awful, agony, unbearable, etc. or from specific questioning and appropriate rating scales.
Duration	Minutes, hours, days.
Aggravating factors	The pain of angina pectoris or intermittent claudication may be associated with exercise, whilst abdominal pain from peptic ulceration may be related to eating habits e.g. being aggravated by hunger and spicy foods. Pleuritic chest pain will be worsened with coughing and deep inspiration.
Relieving factors	The patient may be aware of ways in which the pain may be eased e.g. avoiding coughing, a more comfortable posture, rest, etc.
Times of occurrence	Peptic ulcer may occur in the early hours of the morning; headaches related to raised intracranial pressure will occur in the mornings.
Associated phenomena	Vomiting and visual disturbance may be associated with migraine headaches.
Previous history	Of this or similar pain.

To assess the effectiveness of therapy, a scale such as the following one can be used:

1   No improvement
2   Slight improvement
3   Great improvement
4   No pain

More complicated forms of descriptive scales are available as questionnaires, and these are primarily suitable for research purposes.

Visual analogue scale

This consists of a 10 cm line marked with a phrase such as 'no pain' on the extreme left and 'the worst pain possible' on the extreme right:

No pain _____ The worst pain possible

The patient is asked to draw a line through the scale indicating the severity of the pain. This can then be quantified by measuring the distance from the left of the scale. This is quick to use and relatively simple to understand. It can also be adapted for specific situations such as for children (see Fig. 2.3), when the words are exchanged for pictorial representations such as happy and sad faces. Visual analogue scales can also be easily computerized — the patient moving the cursor along a line on the screen and the distance being automatically measured.

Both descriptive scales and visual analogue scores are primarily designed to be used by patients but they can also both be used by

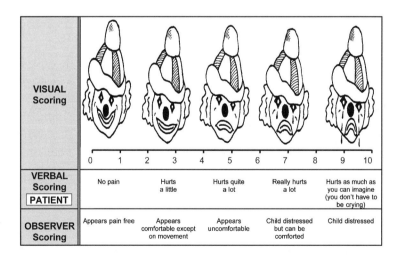

Fig. 2.3 Visual analogue scale adapted for use with children.

an observer. However, this will considerably reduce the accuracy of the assessment. Subjective assessment can also be made, by an observer, of the physiological responses to pain such as pallor, sweating, and behavioural reactions.

2. Objective measurements

These are used less frequently than subjective methods as they are not always applicable and their sensitivity and reproducibility are limited. Many utilize physiological measurements which vary with the severity of pain. Most frequently these are respiratory measurements, which are useful measures after upper abdominal and thoracic operations when pain may limit deep breathing and coughing. Such operations will be accompanied by reductions in arterial oxygen partial pressure, peak expiratory flow rate, and forced vital capacity, along with increases in arterial carbon dioxide partial pressure. Improvements may be correlated with adequate analgesia.

A further objective method of assessing pain is to record the patient's analgesic requirements. For example, to assess the effectiveness of a local anaesthetic block, the patient's opioid requirements before and after the block can be compared.

3

Why treat pain?

The most important reason for treating pain is a basic humanitarian concern; the first requirement of medicine being to alleviate suffering. Good analgesia will reduce patient discomfort and minimize the associated psychological distress. The beneficial effects on several organ systems of better pain control may lead to improved outcome and a reduction in hospital stay. The adverse effects of pain and the stress response to surgery are illustrated in Fig. 3.1.

PULMONARY COMPLICATIONS

Postoperatively, most patients show a major reduction in pulmonary function with lung volumes and flows depressed by 20–60 per cent of preoperative values. This is most obvious in patients who have undergone thoracic and upper abdominal surgery. Coughing and clearing of secretions is markedly impaired when surgery is close to the diaphragm. In addition, since movement results in pain, the diaphragm is held taught and 'splinted'. Gas exchange is abnormal and the development of atelectasis and pneumonia result in significant morbidity.

Early studies looked only at intraoperative anaesthetic techniques — comparing epidural and general anaesthesia — and found no benefit in improved postoperative course. However, the use of continuous epidural local anaesthesia to provide postoperative pain relief showed improvements in pulmonary function and a reduction in pulmonary complications. These techniques have been shown to be better than conventional intramuscular morphine after abdominal and thoracic procedures. Alternative

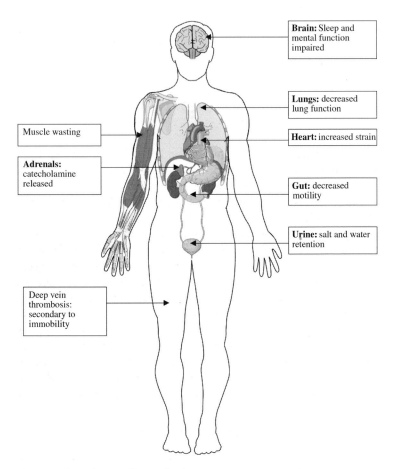

Fig. 3.1 The adverse effects of pain.

local anaesthetic techniques such as intercostal nerve blockade or wound infiltration also produce improvements in postoperative pulmonary function.

Respiratory depression resulting from conventional opioid regimens may be a contributing factor to the development of pulmonary complications after surgery. However, it is clear that an aggressive approach to postoperative pain control can result in measurable improvements in pulmonary function and a reduction in complications. These effects are especially noticeable in high-risk groups such as patients who have had thoracic and upper abdominal operations.

STRESS RESPONSE TO SURGERY AND TRAUMA

There are characteristic endocrine and metabolic changes which occur after surgery, trauma, and infection. These responses have developed from the 'fear, fight, and flight' mechanisms developed to enable the body to survive following injury. The characteristic changes are listed in Table 3.1

In general, increased catabolism is seen with the development of negative nitrogen balance associated with skeletal muscle breakdown. Lipolysis occurs and the patient will exhibit hyperglycaemia and impaired glucose tolerance. As a result of increased sodium and water reabsorption in the kidney, urine output decreases.

Much work is being done to determine whether obtunding the stress response improves outcome. At present the issue is unproven. The two major initiators of the stress response are afferent neuronal impulses and inflammatory mediators released from damaged tissues. The degree of pain felt will also depend on both these factors and may thus be a component in the

Table 3.1 Biochemical and endocrinological changes associated with the stress response to trauma and surgery

Increased pituitary hormone secretion:	↑ β endorphin ↑ ACTH ↑ GH ↑ Prolactin ↑ ADH
Sympathetic nervous system activity:	↑ Adrenaline (epinephrine) ↑ Noradrenaline (norepinephrine)
Fluid and electrolyte changes:	↑ Sodium and water retention ↑ Blood glucose
Skeletal muscle breakdown:	Amino acids used in gluconeogenesis and in the synthesis of acute-phase proteins

initiation of the stress response. It is important to appreciate that the stress response may occur even without perception of pain after surgery.

Variations of anaesthetic techniques and their modifying effects upon the stress response have been studied. Epidural regional anaesthetic techniques have been shown to significantly blunt the stress response following lower abdominal and lower extremity surgery. Systemic opioids are only useful when administered in very high doses. Combinations of regional anaesthetic agents and opioids administered into the epidural space may be beneficial in upper abdominal and thoracic surgery, but may have to be given continuously.

THROMBOEMBOLIC COMPLICATIONS

Virchow described the triad of vascular damage, venous stasis, and hypercoagulability which underlies the development of venous thrombosis. Patients undergoing orthopaedic operations on lower limbs and lower abdominal and pelvic surgery are at particular risk of developing this complication. Pain encourages immobility, resulting in venous stasis, and this increases the risk of deep venous thrombosis.

Epidural anaesthesia and continuous postoperative epidural analgesic techniques reduce the incidence of deep venous thrombosis and may reduce the incidence of pulmonary emboli. It is believed that they do this by both improving the blood flow through the lower limbs by sympathetic blockade and by reducing the hypercoagulable state.

RETURN OF GASTROINTESTINAL FUNCTION

Pain impairs gastrointestinal function and in particular delays gastric emptying. The use of parenteral opioids has also been associated with a reduction in gastrointestinal motility. When epidural analgesia with local anaesthetics alone (without opioids) is used, an earlier return to normal bowel function is seen. This outcome is desirable to maintain adequate nutrition and to reduce hospital stay.

MENTAL STATE

Patients at increased risk of postoperative deterioration of mental function include the elderly. For them, recovery of mental function is particularly important for mobilization and to enable a return to their home environment.

There remains controversy about the influence of anaesthetic drugs and techniques and postoperative analgesia on mental changes. It has been suggested that regional analgesic techniques which reduce or avoid the need for opioid drugs would be of benefit in decreasing the incidence of confusion after operations.

CARDIOVASCULAR FUNCTION

For the patient with heart disease, pain causing hypertension and tachycardia acts as an unnecessary stress on the myocardium. Attention to postoperative analgesia by all methods can be expected to lessen morbidity and mortality by reducing sympathetic drive and catecholamine release.

Thoracic epidural techniques, when used to provide post-operative analgesia, improve myocardial function as a result of sympathetic blockade. This results in reductions in both pre-load and after-load and, in addition, dilation of coronary vessels. This technique can also be of value in patients with crescendo angina that is uncontrolled by other pharmacological means. Improvement is seen not only in pain control but also in myocardial function.

4

Psychological aspects of acute pain

PATIENT FEATURES INFLUENCING PAIN CONTROL

Personality

Emotional state and personality modify our response to pain at the brain level; they do not affect peripheral pain thresholds. The most commonly studied personality traits are extrovertism and neuroticism. Extroverts are believed to complain more about their pain and may receive more analgesics in clinical situations. Patients with high neurotic-scale scores may rate their pain much higher in studies.

Pain is not only associated with the idea of bodily harm but also more complex feelings of guilt, loss, and punishment that may accompany the injury. A patient's strategy for responding to these conflicts may serve to worsen or alleviate the distress. The processes of denial, dissociation, and distraction may help to lessen the pain, whereas patients who catastrophize (characterized by negative attitudes and overly negative thoughts and ideas) will cope less well with their pain. Patients will have acquired these individual strategies from previous experience of pain and their socio-cultural development.

Knowledge and fears relating to the cause, pathology, treatment, and prognosis of their illness, misunderstandings, and inadequate information can lead to increased anxiety in patients. Their distress may be hidden by 'the stiff upper lip' attitude. Recognition and clarification of these problems can reduce the emotional distress.

Anxiety

The influence of anxiety on pain perception and analgesic requirements has also been widely studied. Anxiety can be one of two kinds.

- State anxiety is that which arises from a particular stress and may be anticipatory or situational.
- Trait anxiety is the tendency of an individual to respond to stress with high or low levels of anxiety.

This will be modified by an individual's sociocultural background, early experiences, prior conditioning, and developmental state. High levels of trait anxiety are associated with increased pain perception. Also, even minor levels of depression (which might be considered normal) may influence postoperative pain.

Often obvious differences are seen in the degree and nature of anxiety that patients exhibit. Some will need frequent reassurance and approach all members of staff; others may show unnatural stoicism or a feeling of virtue from suffering.

Patients preparing for surgery often have profound fears about anaesthesia, including the fear of losing control and ultimately of death, and these may be more important than the implications of the operation. Encouragement must be given to broach these fears however irrational they appear. Any previous traumatic anaesthetic or surgical experience must be appreciated so that anxiety may be allayed with sympathetic counselling.

Type of surgery

The type of surgery that the patient is about to undergo is a particularly important factor in preoperative stress. Since the heart is still seen as the physical and emotional centre of life, cardiac surgery is seen, by the patient, as especially threatening. Mutilating operations such as amputations and mastectomy and also some plastic surgery procedures which change body shape are more traumatic psychologically. The well-recognized 'fear of cancer' may be present in many patients before surgery. This may often be an irrational fear (when the patient's symptoms and disease are incompatible with the diagnosis of cancer) and this anxiety may be relieved by careful explanation and reassurance. However, in some cases it may be impossible to reassure the patient until the histological diagnosis is received.

Preoperative discussion with the patient about the effects of their operation and the nature of the pain and other sensations that they will experience following recovery should include the methods available to alleviate pain. It may be too late, at this stage, for instruction in any psychological strategies to be effective.

Information must be presented to each patient in an understandable form. Booklets and videos have been used to prepare patients for hospitalization and surgery, but the patient's hospital attendants must be prepared to reinforce the messages. Many patients will need support and information from all members of staff. Relatives can also offer valuable information and reassurance to the patient.

Children

The young child may have complicated interpretations of illness depending on age and developmental level. Pain control in children has often suffered from the myth that young children do not feel pain or, if they do feel pain, do not remember it. Several factors are important when assessing pain in children:

- developmental level
- parental attitudes
- effects of hospitalization
- symbolic meaning of pain
- physiological response to pain.

The developmental level of a child may limit their ability to communicate that they are in pain. Furthermore, the unknown hospital environment and the child's shyness of strangers may inhibit him or her from asking for pain relief. Young children may perceive injections as assaults and be unable to appreciate that they will relieve pain. Doctors and nurses may overestimate a child's understanding and the effects of illness and hospitalization may also produce regression to earlier developmental levels.

Young children have a special concern about body integrity and fears of possible mutilation. In young children pain may be interpreted as a punishment. Special attention needs to be paid to children's fears when they are prepared for surgery. They can often be helped to adjust to hospital stays by careful preparation including the use of successful techniques such as video or social modelling, behaviour therapies, and hypnosis.

There has been considerable progress over the last 20 years in caring for children in hospital and an increased awareness of their particular problems. Parents are now able to stay with their children and participate in their care. Day-stay surgery allows children to spend shorter periods in hospital and has become increasingly popular.

STRATEGIES FOR THE MANAGEMENT OF PAIN

Pain is a subjective experience which has complex interactions with the emotional state of the patient. The concept of the pain experience as a whole can be considered at three distinct levels.

- The first level is the sensory and discriminative input from the noxious stimulus via the sensory nervous system, for example, the result of sticking your finger with a needle.
- At the second level, motivational factors and the affective state of the patient (awake, asleep, happy, sad) can alter the interpretation of input at the central nervous system.
- Thirdly, the evaluation of the stimulus by our thoughts or cognition, processes the overall response to the pain.

Approaches to the management of pain should therefore be not only directed towards the sensory input but also to emotional and other factors which influence the patient's response. This was described in early work by Beecher (1956*a,b*) and has more recently been developed extensively in pain clinics, for the control of chronic pain.

A trimodal system of pain management has been described where the appropriate therapies available for pain control have been classified into three levels of intervention.

1. Cognitive strategies

Cognitive strategies refer to techniques that influence the pain experience through the medium of thoughts or cognition and they include imagery and attention diversion. These can be taught pre-operatively to patients in preparation for surgery. They have been assessed in volunteers where the studies can be performed before and after the teaching of cognitive controls. In this setting these techniques prolong the ability to withstand previously painful levels of experimental pain. Examples which have been used in these techniques include the following:

Distraction: imagining pleasant events
                     focusing on other things
                     concentrating on sensations other than pain
Dissociation: dissociating from the pain (self hypnosis)
                     imagining the affected area as numb

Perhaps the most common use of psychological strategies to combat pain is in the preparation for childbirth. Behavioural and cognitive techniques are taught to pregnant women to reduce the effects of labour pain. Studies have shown that these techniques provide benefit, particularly in the early stage of labour, although few women can still use these techniques by the time the second stage of labour is reached.

2. Behavioural manipulations

With behavioural strategies, patients exercise a response to the pain, giving them a feeling of control. This element of patient control was first described when nitrous oxide and air mixtures were used to reduce the pain of childbirth. This method recognized the value of allowing patients to control their own analgesia. More recently the introduction of patient-controlled analgesia systems for use with opioid analgesics has highlighted the importance of this.

Other behavioural techniques, which may be useful in both acute and chronic pain, can be divided into two types. A first group, which requires the presence of external people or features to derive the best effects, includes the following.

● Hypnosis.
● Operant conditioning techniques to reinforce helpful pain behaviours.

- Biofeedback training of patients may be useful for recurrent pain problems such as Raynaud's phenomenon and migraine, enabling them to change specific physiological parameters such as skin temperature and muscle tension.
- Modelling techniques: children can be helped by video tapes showing other children's appropriate responses to painful or unpleasant procedures.

A second group, which depends less on external controls, includes the following.

- Placebos: approximately 35 per cent of patients with acute pain will show a response to placebos.
- Perceived controllability: patients who have learnt to feel in control of pain themselves will respond better and report lower pain scores; those who rely on external control will report higher pain scores.

3. Physical intervention

This describes the final level of methods available to influence pain and includes physical and pharmacological interventions.

- Relaxation.
- Physiotherapy: this can include the applications of heat and cold by a variety of means, which may alleviate pain and reduce any associated muscle spasm.
- Transcutaneous nerve stimulation (TENS).
- Acupuncture.
- Pharmacological agents, opioids, non-steroidal anti-inflammatory drugs, and local anaesthetics and inhalational agents.

5
Principles of analgesic drug administration

This section briefly introduces important pharmacological terms which apply to the following chapters on analgesic drug use and administration.

The terms have been subdivided under their respective headings — pharmacokinetic terms and pharmacodynamic terms. Pharmacokinetic terms refer to how the body deals with the drug (that is, how the drug is absorbed, metabolized, and eliminated); pharmacodynamic terms describe the effects of the drug on the body (for example, how the drug binds to its receptor and produces effects).

Pharmacokinetic terms

Bioavailability

This term applies to the percentage of an oral dose which reaches the systemic circulation. It depends upon how much drug is absorbed and the amount of drug undergoing metabolism as it passes through the gut wall or the liver. The term can also be applied to doses given by other routes such as rectal or buccal administration. Knowledge of the bioavailability of drugs allows adjustment of dosages when intravenous drugs are changed to oral preparations and vice versa.

First-pass metabolism

Some drugs, when given orally, may undergo significant metabolism on first pass through the gut wall, liver, or both. This can vary between patients and may be influenced by hepatic blood flow and disease states. There may be up to five-fold increases in plasma drug concentrations in patients with cirrhosis who have porto-systemic shunting because of a reduction in hepatic metabolism of the drug.

The effect of first-pass metabolism means that to produce equivalent effects, an oral dose will need to be considerably greater than a parenteral dose. The degree of first-pass metabolism of a drug will affect its bioavailability.

Clearance

This describes the volume of plasma cleared of the drug in a set time (one minute, for example). It is the result of both hepatic metabolism and renal excretion and elimination by other organs. Knowledge of whether a drug undergoes renal or hepatic clearance allows the appropriate drug to be chosen when dealing with patients in renal or hepatic failure.

Half life

This is defined as the time taken for the plasma concentration of a drug to decrease by half. If after a bolus intravenous injection of a drug, the plasma concentration is measured repeatedly over time a curve such as that in Fig. 5.1 is obtained.

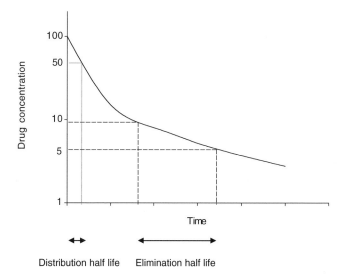

Fig. 5.1 Graph of plasma concentration plotted against time after intravenous bolus of analgesic.

A drug may have two different half lives known as the distribution half life (during which the plasma concentration decreases due to absorption into other body tissues, e.g. fat, muscle) and the elimination half life during which the drug is removed completely from the plasma by metabolism or elimination in bile, urine, etc.

Knowledge of the half life of a drug allows correct dosing intervals to be selected. Morphine has an elimination half life of 1.7–4 hours; remifentanil has an elimination half life of 10–21 minutes. Therefore, bolus doses of remifentanil would need repeating so often to maintain analgesia that in practice it is used only as a continuous infusion.

Pharmacodynamic terms

Agonist

This term applies to an agent, which when combined with a receptor in the body, produces a biological action. Morphine is an opioid receptor (specifically μ receptor) agonist.

Antagonist

This term is used for agents which will block the actions of agonist drugs. Naloxone is a μ receptor antagonist that can reverse the analgesia and side-effects of morphine.

Agonist–antagonist agents

Opioid drugs of this type (for example, meptazinol) have agonist actions at one opioid receptor site and antagonist properties at another. Thus they can also be used as antagonists of pure agonist agents. Some of these agents, as a result of their antagonist properties, can produce symptoms of opioid withdrawal in dependent patients.

Partial agonists

These agents have agonist properties at low doses which do not increase with higher dosages. They have a low intrinsic efficacy and so opioid partial agonists, such as buprenorphine, exhibit a ceiling effect to their analgesic effects.

Dependence

Fear of addiction is often expressed as a concern by people involved in the prescribing and administering of opioids in acute pain. It is an irrational fear and is an important cause of inadequate analgesia being administered to patients in pain. The Boston Collaborative Drug Surveillance Program reviewed the records of 11 882 hospital patients who had received at least one narcotic preparation. Results showed only four reasonably well-documented cases of addiction in patients with no previous history of drug abuse — an incidence of 0.03 per cent.

When opioid drugs are administered for prolonged periods for chronic pain problems they are often restricted to terminal care patients.

Physical dependence

This is demonstrated by the appearance of symptoms and signs of withdrawal (or abstinence) if the drug is abruptly discontinued or opioid antagonists are administered to patients after prolonged opioid use. These effects include sweating, tachycardia, and diarrhoea. The severity of the withdrawal effects is dependent upon the dose and duration of previous opioid administration.

Psychic dependence

This term is used to describe the compulsive drug-seeking behaviour exhibited with addiction. This occurs with opioids, primarily as a result of their mood-altering effects. However, drug use for medical purposes is not a major factor in the development of addiction; when opioids are used to relieve acute pain the development of addiction is rare. Other medical, social, psychological, economic, and cultural factors play important roles in addiction.

Opiate/opioid

The term opiate was originally applied to drugs obtained from opium. These include morphine, codeine, and the semi-synthetic congeners of morphine. Following the development of totally synthetic drugs with morphine-like actions, the term opioid was developed. It now stands as the generic designation for all exogenous substances that bind to any of the several subtypes of opioid receptors and produce agonist actions. However, in many texts the terms opioid and opiate are used interchangeably.

Potency

The response to a drug is usually plotted on a dose–response curve. A variety of drugs with the same actions can be compared using these graphs. The most potent drug will produce its pharmacological effects at lower doses. However, the low potency of an individual drug may be overcome by increasing the dosage used.

Tolerance

The development of tolerance is seen after a drug has been administered for some time and a given dose of drug produces a decreasing effect. Thus larger doses of the drug are required to produce the original level of effect. With opioid analgesics the first indication of tolerance may be a reduction in the duration of effect. As tolerance to analgesia develops, so too does tolerance to the sedative and respiratory depressant effects of opioids. However, tolerance to the smooth-muscle effects of opioids, for example constipation, is slow to develop. Fortunately, with acute pain, in the majority of patients, pain will be decreasing over the time that tolerance develops.

PHARMACOLOGICAL FACTORS IMPORTANT IN ANALGESIC DRUG ADMINISTRATION

Changes in the effects of drugs may follow changes in the concentration of drug available at the site of action resulting from altered pharmacokinetics. Alternatively, individual sensitivity to drugs may result from alterations at the receptor level where the drug acts (pharmacodynamics). Disease states may also predispose to changes in sensitivity brought about by alterations in receptor sensitivity.

Age also affects many of the variables already mentioned, resulting in increased sensitivity to many drugs in the elderly patient. With analgesic drugs, hepatic metabolism and renal excretion may be reduced and also altered receptor sensitivity may be responsible for reduced drug requirements. Neonates and infants under six months have increased sensitivity to the depressant effects of opioids. Reduced hepatic metabolism and increased permeability of the blood–brain barrier to drugs may be responsible.

When an analgesic drug is administered, the amount remaining in the body at any given time will depend on the following:

- Route of administration
- Frequency of administration
- Rate of release of the drug from its formulation
- Rate of absorption from the site of administration
- The amount of metabolism that occurs in the gut wall or liver as the drug is absorbed (first-pass metabolism)
- The rate of distribution to organs and tissues
- Routes and rates of metabolism
- Routes and rates of excretion

In any individual patient, disease states may also alter any of these factors.

ROUTES OF ADMINISTRATION OF ANALGESIC DRUGS

In clinical practice several routes are available for analgesic administration. These are discussed in this chapter. For a comparison of the various drug administration routes available see Table 5.1

Parenteral routes of drug administration

Intravenous injection

The intravenous route is the most important route for analgesic drug administration in the treatment of acute pain. Its advantages include the immediate access of the drug to the circulation, ensuring 100% bioavailability and rapid onset of action. It may be used for single intravenous doses (bolus) or for continuous infusion.

There are disadvantages with this route which include the need to secure intravenous access (and the maintenance of this access for prolonged periods), the need for medical staff or specially trained nurses to be available to administer intravenous boluses, and the possibility that the drug may be more rapidly eliminated, thereby shortening its duration of action.

Table 5.1 Advantages and disadvantages of the various routes available for analgesic drug administration

Route	Advantage	Disadvantage
Oral	No injections needed Easily administered	Fasting, post-gastrointestinal surgery patients not suitable Nausea and vomiting reduce reliability of this route Unpredictable absorption and bioavailability of drugs Requires conscious or co-operative patient or nasogastric tube
Intravenous	Rapid onset 100% bioavailability Suitable for continuous infusion techniques	Venous access required Nursing/medical staff required to give drugs High-peak plasma concentrations achieved easily and may cause side-effects
Intramuscular	Standard route used in wards Relatively rapid onset of analgesia	Intermittent technique Painful injections Risk of nerve/vascular damage Variable absorption e.g. in shock
Subcutaneous	Relatively easy access Small cannulae can be used for repeated injections	Variable absorption e.g. in shock Irritant and painful injections Risk of abscess and infection Depot of drug may remain in skin even after infusions stopped
Sublingual/buccal	Bypasses first-pass metabolism Independent of gastric emptying or vomiting High patient acceptability	Patient co-operation needed to prevent chewing/swallowing of preparation Slow saliva production reduces dissolution of tablets Taste important for acceptance

Route	Advantage	Disadvantage
Rectal	Reduced first-pass metabolism Useful for slow-release preparations of drugs Independent of gastric emptying or vomiting	Low patient acceptance Slow absorption and slow onset of effect Unpredictable bioavailability
Transdermal	Slow-release preparations useful for background analgesia	Few drugs available Depot remains in skin after preparation removed Slow onset and offset of analgesia Difficult to titrate against acute pain
Inhalational (nitrous oxide)	Rapid onset and offset of effects Moderately potent analgesic Useful for episodic pain of short duration	Bone marrow depression with prolonged use (>12 h) Pollution of working environment Patient co-operation required
Epidural and spinals (see Chapter 14)	Excellent prolonged analgesia possible with infusions Minimal sedation Minimal impairment of respiratory function	Technically challenging to site Requires close nursing observations for rare but serious adverse effects

Intramuscular injection

This is the commonest parenteral route used for the administration of opioid analgesic drugs on hospital wards. The standard prescription for analgesia is for intramuscular injections of an opioid given four-hourly as required. This has many disadvantages. The patient must express a demand for analgesia; few patients can anticipate the end of the analgesic effect of the drugs and will therefore be in pain before each demand is met. In addition, a standard time of four hours between doses may be too long for healthy, young adults but be too short a time interval for elderly patients. It has gained acceptance because it does not require medical supervision for its administration and is simple to give.

When administered by this route the rate of absorption of the drugs is dependent upon muscle blood flow. The onset of effects will therefore be slower than after intravenous injection. Additional disadvantages include the pain caused by the injections and the risks of major bruising in patients with coagulation problems. Injections at inappropriate sites in the buttocks and thigh have been known to result in vascular and neural damage.

Subcutaneous injection

The subcutaneous route provides an accessible parenteral route for the administration of analgesic drugs. The absorption of drug from the subcutaneous site is dependent upon regional skin blood flow and this may make it unsuitable for use in patients where skin perfusion is reduced, particularly the shocked, hypovolaemic patient. More recently, the use of small cannulae placed subcutaneously has allowed this route to be used for repeated intermittent dosing or for continuous infusion of drugs.

Drugs administered subcutaneously may be irritant and the injection can be painful. In some cases abscess formation may occur.

Oral

This is the standard route of administration for most drugs. However, this route is often not practicable when treating acute pain. Pain itself reduces gastric emptying, making this route ineffective. Postoperative vomiting and gastrointestinal stasis will also render the oral route unsuitable. In the uncooperative or unconscious patient, the oral route will not be available, although some patients may have a nasogastric tube in place which may be used.

The need to achieve analgesia rapidly in the distressed patient is of considerable importance. Drugs given by the oral route are dependent upon the physical dissolution of the drug formulation, the rate of gastric emptying, and gastrointestinal motility before absorption takes place through the mucosa of the small intestine. The rate of gastric emptying and gastrointestinal motility may be delayed postoperatively or as a result of opioid administration, therefore limiting its use. However, the use of an oral slow-release preparation of analgesic, perhaps administered preoperatively, may be helpful in providing analgesia in the early postoperative period.

Suitable drugs include slow-release morphine or some non-steroidal anti-inflammatory analgesics. The opioid drugs, in particular, are subject to extensive first-pass metabolism when given by the oral route and the doses required to produce equivalent analgesia are considerably greater than by parenteral routes. Three to six times the dose of morphine may be required to be given orally as compared with the intramuscular route to produce equivalent effects.

Commonly, acute pain gradually improves over a period of 2–3 days. Initially, patients may require parenteral therapy with opioid analgesics, but as requirements for analgesia reduce, the patient may be managed with oral opioids, non-steroidal anti-inflammatory drugs, or combinations of these drugs, providing gastrointestinal absorption is adequate.

Epidural and intrathecal

Following the discovery of the opioid receptors in the substantia gelatinosa of the spinal cord, the direct application of opioid drugs to this area was investigated and has proved successful in producing analgesia. Local anaesthetic agents may also be administered by these routes to provide analgesia. The use of the epidural and intrathecal routes of administration in analgesia have increased. The theory, applications, and complications of these routes of administration are discussed in Chapter 14.

Non-parenteral routes of drug administration

To overcome the inability to use the oral route to provide analgesia, alternative non-parenteral routes of administration including sublingual, buccal, rectal, transdermal, and intranasal may be utilized.

Sublingual/buccal

The advantages of these routes include avoiding first-pass metabolism of drugs and the need for injections. Drug absorption remains independent of gastric emptying, vomiting, and gastrointestinal motility. They are acceptable to patients because they escape the pain of injections — although some co-operation is required to prevent the chewing or swallowing of the drug preparation. Drugs can be formulated as a tablet, solution, or paste. The form influences the rate of absorption through the oral mucous membranes. Absorption through the buccal mucosa of some opioids is rapid and because first-pass metabolism is avoided, most of the drug is available for analgesia.

Taste is obviously important in patient acceptance of these routes of administration. Many of the opioids produce a bitter taste when given sublingually or buccally, thus limiting their use. Problems may occur with both of these routes in patients with reduced saliva production, which makes dissolution of tablet preparations slow. Some drug will be lost by chewing and swallowing even with good patient co-operation. If there is delayed gastric emptying, this may produce a considerable depot of analgesic drug in the stomach, which may be rapidly absorbed once gastrointestinal function is restored.

Rectal

This is a further route which utilizes the end portion of the gastrointestinal tract without the disadvantages of oral administration. The use of the rectal route has not gained wide patient acceptance in British medical practice, although it enjoys popularity in other countries. Slow absorption of the drug preparation leads to a slow onset of analgesia which is a disadvantage in the initial management of acute pain. Although first-pass metabolism is reduced, the amount of drug that is available for analgesic purposes is variable.

The rectal route is well suited to the maintenance of analgesia and slow-release preparations are often used. It is sometimes used during anaesthesia as a route for NSAIDs.

Transdermal

This is a new technique and few analgesic drugs are available at present. For a drug to be used transdermally, it must ideally be lipid soluble (to pass through stratum corneum) and water soluble (to pass through the dermis), have a high potency (so that a therapeutic dose can pass through a small area of skin), be non-irritant to the skin, and not be metabolized by the skin. As the blood flow to the skin and hence drug absorption can vary depending on the degree and type of thermal stress, a membrane is incorporated into the drug delivery system to act as a limiting step in the rate of drug delivery. The rate of drug delivered is directly proportional to the size of the patch.

A transdermal fentanyl preparation is currently available but is not recommended or approved for acute pain. Studies conducted in the acute pain setting raised fears of clinically significant respiratory depression and the slow changes in plasma concentrations (steady state not reliably reached after 24 hours) made titrating doses to constantly changing acute postoperative pain very difficult. Transdermal fentanyl has however been used to manage the long-standing, less variable pain of cancer.

Intranasal

Midazolam and fentanyl have both been used via this route. In a study in acute postoperative pain using metered fentanyl nasal sprays delivering 27 µg each time, analgesia almost equivalent to intravenous fentanyl was achieved within 10 minutes. Thus it has been suggested as a means of analgesia after intravenous cannulae have been removed or for breakthrough pain in cancer.

6

Opioid pharmacology

Opioid agents have effects on many systems in the body. This chapter describes some of these effects. Figure 6.1 summarizes these effects.

CENTRAL NERVOUS SYSTEM EFFECTS

Opioid agents have a variety of effects on the central nervous system, which can be broadly classified as depressant or excitatory.

Depressant effects

Analgesia

This is the most common indication for the therapeutic use of opioid drugs. It results from the action of opioids at a number of levels in the central nervous system:

1. They have direct effects at spinal cord level in the dorsal horn region.
2. They may influence the descending inhibitory pathways in the brain stem.
3. They have mood-elevating effects acting through the limbic system.

Respiratory depression

Depression of the respiratory centres found in the medulla have a reduced response to carbon dioxide. A slow respiratory pattern, with large tidal volumes, is characteristic of opioid-induced respiratory depression.

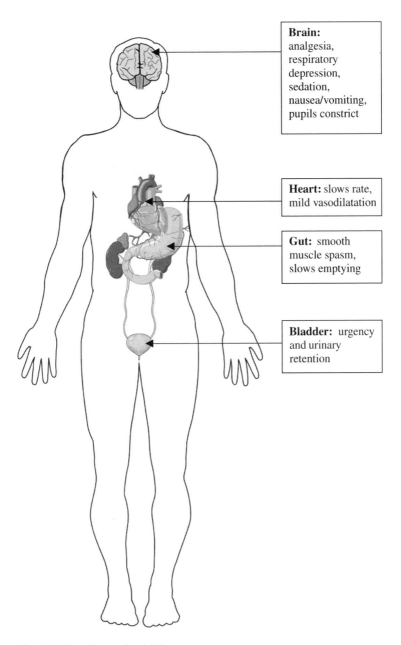

Brain: analgesia, respiratory depression, sedation, nausea/vomiting, pupils constrict

Heart: slows rate, mild vasodilatation

Gut: smooth muscle spasm, slows emptying

Bladder: urgency and urinary retention

Fig. 6.1 The effects of opioids on some organs.

Sedation

Drowsiness is a common feature of opioid use. It may be due to the direct effect of opioids and also to the relief of pain and reduced perception of external stimuli. Occasionally euphoriant properties predominate, resulting from a paradoxical excitation usually due to depression of central inhibitory pathways.

Cough suppression (antitussive effects)

This was a previously widely used indication for opioid therapy and this effect of opioids is still relevant for patients needing ventilatory support. Suppression of coughing results from the action of opioids on medullary cough centres. It is not a universal property of opioids but appears to be related to particular chemical configurations as codeine and diamorphine are more effective than morphine. The antitussive effects of the opioid drugs may be a useful adjunct to their analgesic effects in intubated, critically ill patients by helping them tolerate the tracheal tube.

Excitatory effects

Pupillary constriction

All opioids stimulate the Edinger–Westphal nucleus of the occulomotor nerve, resulting in miosis.

Nausea and vomiting

This may result from a combination of opioid drug effects. There is direct stimulation of the chemoreceptor trigger zone and the vomiting centre situated in the medulla and brain stem. These effects are potentiated by vestibular stimulation, hence the worsening of nausea and vomiting once patients become more mobile.

CARDIOVASCULAR EFFECTS

In normal therapeutic doses the cardiovascular effects of opioids are minimal. Bradycardia may be seen with morphine and fentanyl, whereas pethidine has weak atropine-like effects resulting in a slight increase in heart rate. Vasodilatation, as a result of depression of the medullary vasomotor centres, may occur. In addition, morphine has a direct vasodilatory effect on blood vessels.

GASTROINTESTINAL EFFECTS

Opioids cause contraction of smooth muscle throughout the gastrointestinal tract; gastric emptying is delayed, intestinal transit time is prolonged, and there may be spasm of the anal sphincter.

A well-recognized but infrequent problem is the production of symptoms suggestive of biliary colic after opioid administration. These occur as a result of spasm of the biliary tree and sphincter of Oddi and an increase in intrabiliary pressure. Pethidine does not cause the same increase in intrabiliary pressure as does morphine, although its effects on biliary spasm are still significant. These properties have led to the use of pethidine as the first-line opioid analgesic for the pain of biliary colic.

URINARY TRACT EFFECTS

The detrusor muscle in the bladder and urinary sphincter at the exit of the bladder may contract in response to opioids, leading to urgency and inability to void. Urinary retention is more common in men. It is a frequent problem after the epidural administration of opioids.

HISTAMINE RELEASE

Allergic responses to opioids are extremely rare. Morphine, pethidine, and codeine are all known to release histamine, which may result in vasodilatation. Manifestations of histamine release which may be seen include: erythema, pruritis, urticaria, and bronchospasm. Codeine is not given intravenously as profound hypotension results secondary to histamine release.

Symptoms resulting from allergic reactions to opioids may include sweating, nausea, chest pain, and palpitations. Transient loss of consciousness may occur as a result of hypotension. In patients who have allergic reactions to opioids there may be some cross sensitivity between individual agents.

RESPIRATORY EFFECTS

The clinical significance of respiratory depression

Excessive amounts of opioids cause a decrease in respiratory rate and conscious level which can result in hypercarbia (high carbon dioxide levels in the blood). Coma may result as carbon dioxide has narcotic properties itself. Coma in turn may progress to apnoea, hypoxia, and death. However, unrealistic fear of this complication is a major impediment to adequate pain control. Warning signs are seen well in advance of the situation becoming dangerous. With careful monitoring of patients receiving opioids the problem can be minimized.

The respiratory depressant effects of opioids vary, not only with different agents, but also with the same agent given by different routes of administration. Synergy between local anaesthetics and opioids given epidurally or intrathecally will decrease the dose of opioid needed. This may decrease the incidence of respiratory depression when compared to an equianalgesic dose of intravenous or intramuscular opioids. However, when these effects do occur after spinal administration they may be delayed for up to 4–24 hours later.

The use of intravenous infusions of opioids may provide improved analgesia but when compared with standard intermittent intramuscular injections this technique is associated with increased episodes of slow respiratory rates and apnoea. Similarly, postoperative analgesic methods using opioids when compared with those using local-anaesthetic techniques result in increased episodes of arterial oxygen desaturation, indicating intermittent respiratory insufficiency. These episodes occur most commonly when patients are asleep, which appears to have an additive effect on opioid-induced respiratory depression. Supplemental oxygen will reduce the incidence of arterial desaturation, but abnormalities of respiratory rate and apnoea will persist.

Monitoring patients being given opioids

For most patients on the general ward receiving opioids the respiratory rate, level of sedation, and the pain score are monitored. Respiratory rates under 9 breaths per minute (whether asleep or awake) should cause concern. Such patients should either have their dose of opiates reduced or be transferred to a critical care area for closer monitoring. Intermittent monitoring of respiratory rate alone will not detect transient events or apnoeic episodes after opioid therapy. Furthermore, some patients may have normal respiratory rates but still be hypoxic or hypercarbic. If other measurements such as pulse and blood pressure, which disturb the patient, are combined with respiratory rate measures, then true resting effects will not be monitored. Sedation scoring in combination with respiratory rate allows the earlier detection of excess opiate administration.

Pulse oximetry allows the oxygen saturation of haemoglobin to be monitored noninvasively whereas arterial blood gases and transcutaneous electrodes allow the partial pressure of oxygen and carbon dioxide to be monitored.

The pulse oximeter is the best indirect method available for monitoring arterial oxygen saturation (SaO_2). This equipment uses the differential absorption of light by saturated and desaturated haemoglobin to produce a continuous display of pulse rate and oxygen saturation. Sensors are comfortable for the patients and can be used for long-term monitoring. The equipment has a rapid response time to changing saturations. Normal saturation levels are of the order of 95–99% (equivalent to a partial pressure of oxygen in arterial blood (PaO_2) of greater than 10 KPa) and the equipment is accurate to low saturations of 70% (PaO_2 under 7 KPa). Pulse oximetry is useful in detecting hypoxia which occurs only when carbon dioxide levels are very high in the lungs (i.e. relatively late in respiratory depression caused by opioids). If the patient is on oxygen, the pulse oximeter may not show low saturations even when the patient is comatose.

Transcutaneous measurements of PaO_2 and $PaCO_2$ have proved reliable in children and have been widely used in neonatal intensive care. Their use in adults is difficult, as variations in skin thickness influence the results. The sensors heat up the skin resulting in the need for frequent changes of site to reduce the risk of burns, particularly in the small premature infant.

In patients who are at high risk of developing respiratory complications (e.g. in those with chest injuries or following thoracic and upper-abdominal surgery in patients with pre-existing pulmonary disease) indwelling arterial cannula allows frequent sampling for arterial blood–gas analysis. Arterial canulae are only used in intensive care units or in operating theatres.

The partial pressure of carbon dioxide in the blood rises whenever ventilation is inadequate (whatever the cause) or falls if ventilation is excessive. The partial pressure of carbon dioxide is a better indicator of ventilatory adequacy than partial pressure of oxygen.

The use of naloxone to treat respiratory depression is described on page 67 (Chapter 7).

7

Useful opioid analgesic drugs

The analgesic and euphoric properties of opium have been known for several thousand years. The word 'opium' is derived from the Greek, meaning juice — the source of the juice being the unripe seed-heads of the poppy *Papaver somniferum*. Despite the years of use and abuse its derivatives still remain a useful and rightly popular drug for the treatment of pain.

PROPERTIES OF AN IDEAL OPIOID

The ideal agent for analgesic use should have:

- rapid onset of analgesic effect;
- no accumulation following prolonged administration;
- safe and reliable elimination even with impaired hepatic or renal function;
- lack of acute or chronic toxicity, enzyme induction, or tachyphylaxis;
- no depression of respiration;
- cardiovascular stability;
- no adverse endocrinological effects;
- no increase in muscle tone;
- no venous irritation;
- high therapeutic ratio (a large difference between therapeutic and toxic dose);
- lack of active metabolites;
- simple administration by all routes — intramuscular (IM), intravenous (IV), subcutaneous, oral;
- no addictive potential;

- no absorption on to plastic or glass;
- no interactions with other drugs;
- water solubility, so that the effects of solvents can be ignored;
- stability in solution and on exposure to light, allowing easy storage;
- low cost;
- the same bioavailability when given by all routes so that drug dosage does not depend on route of administration.

CURRENTLY USED DRUGS

Table 7.1 lists the dosage equivalents of opioids discussed in this and the subsequent chapter.

Table 7.1 Equianalgesic IM doses of commonly used opioids for a 70 kg adult

Opioid	Equianalgesic doses	Dose interval
Morphine	10 mg IM	3–4 h
Papaveretum	20 mg IM	3–4 h
Diamorphine	5 mg IM	3–4 h
Pethidine	100 mg IM	3–4 h
Buprenorphine	0.3–0.6 mg IM	6–8 h
Methadone	10 mg IM	8–12 h

Pure agonist drugs

Morphine

Morphine was originally identified by Serturner, a German chemist, in 1805. It is the standard agent against which the activity of all other analgesics may be measured and remains the most valuable opioid analgesic. Its chemical structure is shown in Fig. 7.1. Early attempts at modification of the morphine molecule led to the synthesis of diamorphine and hydromorphone and the discovery of codeine.

In the treatment of acute, severe pain, morphine may be given intravenously or intramuscularly. The standard dose is 10–15

58

mg/70 kg repeated four-hourly intramuscularly. When given intra-venously, smaller doses of 2–5 mg should be given and repeated after 5–10 min until adequate analgesia has been obtained. Opioid drugs are generally not recommended for infants under six months, unless they are in an intensive-care environment, as this group appear to be extremely sensitive to the respiratory-depressant

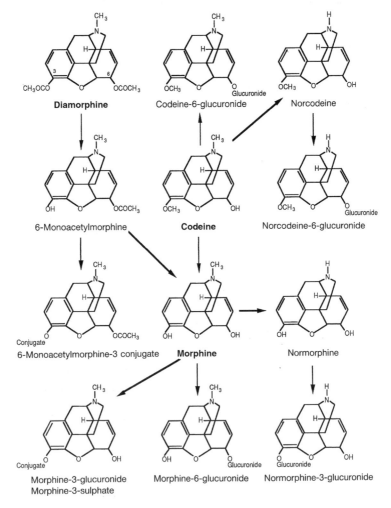

Fig. 7.1 Chemical structures of morphine, diamorphine, and codeine, and their metabolites.

effects. The recommended dose of morphine for older children is 0.15–0.2 mg/kg.

Oral preparations of morphine are available; however, morphine undergoes significant first-pass metabolism. When morphine is given orally, 20–30 mg is equivalent to 10 mg given by the intra-muscular route. New oral preparations of morphine (Sevredol, Napp Laboratories Ltd) may prove useful in the management of acute pain.

The duration of effective analgesia obtained from morphine is approximately three hours.

Adult doses:	2–5 mg IV
	5–15 mg IM
	30–40 mg oral
Children:	0.02 mg/kg IV
	0.2 mg/kg IM
Onset of action:	15–20 min IM
	5–10 min IV
Duration of action:	3 h

Morphine is metabolized principally in the liver to morphine 3-glucuronide and morphine 6-glucuronide. A small proportion is excreted unchanged via the kidney. The metabolite morphine 6-glucuronide is also pharmacologically active and may accumulate in patients with renal failure.

Papaveretum

This agent is a mixture of alkaloids consisting of 253 parts morphine, 23 parts papaverine and 20 parts codeine hydrochloride. Like pethidine, it has a spasmolytic effect that morphine lacks. It is available in two strengths, as 7.7 mg/ml and 15.4 mg/ml which should be clearly specified on the prescription.

It is not recommended for women in the childbearing age group.

7.7 mg of papaveretum is equivalent to 5 mg of morphine.

Adult doses:	7.7–15.4 mg/4 hourly SC, IV, IM
Children:	0.11–0.23 mg/kg SC, IV or IM
Onset of action:	15–20 min IM
	5–10 min IV
Duration of action:	3 h

Diamorphine

The chemical structure of diamorphine is shown in Fig. 7.1. It differs from the structure of morphine in that the two hydroxyl groups in positions 3 and 6 are replaced by acetyl groups. These increase the lipid solubility of diamorphine, which allows it to penetrate rapidly into brain tissue. Once administered the diamorphine is rapidly de-acetylated to produce 6-monoacetyl morphine, which rapidly diffuses into the brain, and is finally converted to morphine. These metabolites are responsible for the analgesic effects of diamorphine.

Diamorphine is available in both oral and parenteral preparations. Its high degree of solubility, allowing high concentrations to be available in small volumes, is an asset.

When given by intramuscular injection, peak plasma concentrations are obtained within 10 minutes. After intravenous administration the drug is quickly distributed producing a more rapid onset of action in comparison to morphine. It is used parenterally for the treatment of acute pain of many forms and has been used to provide analgesia after myocardial infarction.

5 mg of diamorphine is equivalent to 10 mg of morphine.

Adult doses:	2–5 mg IM or IV
Children:	0.1 mg/kg IM
Onset of action:	5–10 min IM
	2–5 min IV
Duration of action:	3 h

Methadone

This is a synthetic opioid with a prolonged duration of action and slow elimination. It undergoes little first-pass metabolism when administered by the oral route. The duration of analgesia is of the order of 6–8 hours. However, accumulation will occur with frequent doses due to its prolonged elimination half life.

10 mg of methadone IM is equivalent to 10 mg of morphine. Oral doses of 10–15 mg are equianalgesic with oral doses of morphine in the range of 40–60 mg.

Adult doses:	5–10 mg IM
Children:	not recommended
Onset of action:	10–15 min IM
	30–60 min oral
Duration of action:	6–8 h

Pethidine

This drug is a synthetic opioid agonist which is a phenylpiperidine derivative. It undergoes rapid metabolism in the liver by microsomal oxidation and is therefore subject to extensive first-pass metabolism when given orally. One of its metabolites, norpethidine, is a central nervous system stimulant and may accumulate in patients with impaired renal function or in patients receiving prolonged infusions of pethidine, resulting in convulsions.

In comparison to other opioids, pethidine does not produce bradycardia by virtue of its atropine-like effects at cholinergic nerve endings.

Drug interaction: if pethidine is given to patients receiving monoamine oxidase inhibitors, central nervous system excitation and hypertension or hypotension may occur.

100 mg of pethidine is equivalent to 10 mg of morphine.

Adult doses:	10–20 mg IV (repeated as necessary)
	50–150 mg IM
	50–300 mg oral
Children:	1 mg/kg IV
	1.5–2 mg/kg IM
Onset of action:	10–15 min IM
	15–30 min oral
Duration of action:	2 h

Phenoperidine

This drug is a synthetic opioid agonist that is chemically related to pethidine. It is most frequently used as an adjunct to anaesthesia or in intensive care units for its analgesic and respiratory depressant effects in patients requiring mechanical ventilation. Unwanted central nervous system effects may be seen in patients with renal failure when phenoperidine may be metabolized to pethidine and subsequently to norpethidine, which will accumulate.

2 mg of phenoperidine is equivalent to 10 mg of morphine.

Adult doses: 0.5–1 mg IV
Children: 30–50 µg/kg

In patients receiving assisted ventilation, doses of 1–2 mg (adults) or 100–150 µg/kg (children) may be repeated.

Onset of action: 2 min IV
Duration of action: 40–60 min

Fentanyl and derivatives

These drugs are newer synthetic opioid agonists that are chemically related to pethidine. In general they are drugs with a short duration of action. They are most commonly used during anaesthesia and for critically ill patients requiring intensive care. Due to their potency they should only be prescribed by the medical staff working in these disciplines.

Fentanyl

There is little cardiovascular depression with this drug although a vagally mediated slowing of heart rate may occasionally be seen. It may also be administered into the epidural space to provide analgesia (see Chapter 17). Higher doses than those given may be required in critically ill patients receiving assisted ventilation.

100 µg of fentanyl is equivalent to 10 mg of morphine.

Adult doses: 50–200 µg IV
Children: 1–3 µg/kg IV
Onset of action: 1–2 min IV
Duration of action: 30–60 min

Alfentanil

Alfentanil has a rapid onset of action with a very short duration of effect. It is often used as a perioperative analgesic agent for patients undergoing outpatient surgical procedures because of its short action and rapid rate of metabolism. Its rapid metabolism has led to it being used in infusion systems, providing analgesia with low risk of drug accumulation.

1 mg of alfentanil is equivalent to 10 mg of morphine.

Adult doses:	Initially up to 500 µg IV
Children:	Initially 10–50 µg/kg IV
Onset of action:	1–2 min IV
Duration of action:	15–20 min

Remifentanil

Remifentanil is a new opioid that is eliminated uniquely by hydrolysis by non-specific esterases. The enzymes that metabolize it are found in large amounts in all tissues and, therefore, remifentanil does not accumulate even after prolonged infusions. Because of this method of metabolism, it is very short acting and needs to be given by infusion. It also wears off very quickly once the infusion is stopped, within 2 to 5 minutes. The very short duration of action and potent respiratory depression it induces also limits its use to the duration of an anaesthetic. If it is used as the sole analgesic and the infusion is switched off at the end of an anaesthetic, when the patient awakens, they have no analgesia and may be in severe pain. Appropriate analgesia must therefore be started before the infusion of remifentanil is stopped. This may be an intravenous dose of morphine, a NSAID, or an epidural top-up.

Currently, remifentanil is being used to provide intraoperative analgesia for cardiac, abdominal, and other forms of surgery. Though novel uses are being explored, it is unlikely to be used on the general ward or in the accident and emergency department owing to its potent side-effects.

100 µg of remifentanil is equianalgesic to 10 mg morphine.

Adult infusion regime: in ventilated patients, 0.05–2 µg/kg/min titrated to response.

Codeine

This drug is unusual as an opioid agonist in that it still retains high oral efficacy owing to low first-pass metabolism. Approximately 10 per cent of the dose is metabolized to morphine and this may be the source of its analgesic properties. The route of metabolism is by an enzyme that is lacking in 10 per cent of the population; in them poor analgesia will result from codeine administration. The remainder of the dose is metabolized to codeine-6-glucuronide.

Codeine itself has a low affinity for the μ receptors. Codeine is not given intravenously as this results in profound histamine release.

120 mg of codeine IM is equianalgesic to 10 mg morphine.

Adult doses:	30–60 mg IM
	30–60 mg oral
Children:	3 mg/kg IM, PO, or PR daily in divided doses.
Onset of action:	30–60 min orally
	10–15 min IM
Duration of action:	4–6 h

Dihydrocodeine

This agent is of similar structure and potency to codeine and may be given orally or intramuscularly.

60 mg is equivalent to 10 mg morphine IM.

Adult doses:	50 mg IM
	30 mg oral
Children:	0.5–1 mg/kg.
Onset of action:	30–60 min orally
	15–20 min IM
Duration of action:	4–5 h

As a result of their oral efficacy, codeine and dihydrocodeine are often used in the management of moderate pain when parenteral administration is unnecessary.

Tramadol

Tramadol is a synthetic opioid with analgesic potency equivalent to pethidine and is used in the management of severe to moderate pain. It differs from the other opioids by inhibiting central neuronal uptake of noradrenaline (norepinephrine) and enhancing serotonin release in addition to being an opioid receptor agonist . In this way it is thought to enhance descending inhibitory pathways as well as inhibiting ascending pain pathways (like conventional opioids). Its use has been limited by side-effects of nausea and vomiting.

The advantages of the drug are that it seems to cause less respiratory depression after intravenous administration in an equipotent dose to morphine and is not subject to controlled drug regulations.

100mg of tramadol is equipotent to 10mg morphine.

Adult dose:	50–100 mg; 4-6 hourly; IV, IM, or oral
Children:	Not recommended

Partial agonist drugs

Buprenorphine

This drug is a semi-synthetic derivative of thebaine, an alkaloid of opium. It is a partial agonist at the μ receptor. Although it has a high affinity for the μ receptor it has a low intrinsic efficacy. It is rapidly absorbed after intramuscular injection or sublingual administration and peak plasma concentrations are found within five minutes of the intramuscular dose.

Respiratory depression may be seen with buprenorphine. This is not readily reversed by naloxone (the specific opioid antagonist) and the use of a non-specific respiratory stimulant, such as doxapram, or ventilatory support, may be needed. Side-effects including sweating, nausea and vomiting, and dizziness can be troublesome.

0.4 mg IM is equianalgesic with 10 mg morphine.

Adult doses:	0.4–0.8 mg sublingual
	0.3–0.6 mg IM
Onset of action:	5 min IM/sublingual
Duration of action:	6–8 h

Agonist–antagonist drugs

Pentazocine

This drug is a synthetic opioid with a benzomorphan structure and is a weak μ antagonist and κ agonist. It exhibits a ceiling effect to its analgesic actions and also to its respiratory-depressant effects.

30 mg is equivalent to 10 mg IM morphine. 50 mg orally is equivalent to 60 mg of codeine.

Adult doses:	30–60 mg IM
	25–50 mg oral
Children:	1 mg/kg IM, 0.5 mg/kg IV
Onset of action:	15 min IM
	1 h oral
Duration of action:	3–4 h

Nalbuphine

The analgesic effects of this agent result from its κ-agonist activity. Structurally it is related to naloxone and oxymorphone. It exhibits marked antagonistic activity at μ receptors. The ceiling effect on respiratory depression is also seen. Dysphoria is less common unless high doses are used.

10 mg IM is equianalgesic with 10 mg morphine.

Adult doses: 10 mg IM/IV
Children: 300 μg/kg IM/IV
Onset of action: 10–15 min IM
Duration of action: 3–4 h

Meptazinol

This drug is also an agonist–antagonist combination and it is reputed to have a low incidence of respiratory depression in therapeutic doses. Nausea and vomiting are its principal adverse effects. Its use has been advocated in obstetrics as an alternative analgesic to pethidine for pain relief in labour.

100 mg IM is equianalgesic to 10 mg morphine.

Adult doses: 75–100 mg IM
                       200 mg oral
Children: not recommended
Onset of action: 15 min IM
                       1 h oral
Duration of action: 3–4 h, with reports of up to 7 h

Opioid antagonist drugs

Naloxone

This is the only agent in general use. It is a competitive antagonist at the μ, δ, and κ receptors. Opioid antagonists will also block the analgesic response to placebo and also that obtained from the low-frequency acupuncture stimulation. It is thought that these effects are mediated through blockade of the endogenous opioid peptide systems. Naloxone also reverses the psychotomimetic and dysphoric effects of opioid drugs but higher doses are required (10–15 mg). Naloxone is ineffective if given orally as it undergoes extensive first-pass metabolism in the liver.

Small doses of naloxone (see following section) will rapidly reverse respiratory depression. Sedation is reversed and an increase in respiratory rate may be seen within 1–2 minutes. Sudden reversal of analgesia is not without risk: vomiting, emergence delirium, dysrhythmias, and pulmonary oedema have been reported in patients after surgery. These unwanted effects may result from a sudden outpouring of catecholamines such as adrenaline (epinephrine) when analgesia is rapidly reversed. Naloxone will also precipitate an intense withdrawal state in patients who are physically dependent on opioids.

Naloxone and management of respiratory depression

When given to patients who have opioid-induced respiratory depression, 0.4 mg of naloxone should be diluted in 10 ml of 0.9 per cent saline and given in divided doses. Doses of 1 ml should be given over a period of 15 seconds and repeated. Once the respiratory depression is reversed no further naloxone should be administered. Naloxone is metabolized in the liver and has a short duration of action of around 30 minutes to 1 hour. The latter means that repeated bolus doses of naloxone may be needed and these may be given intramuscularly or subcutaneously if necessary.

Naltrexone

This drug is an opioid antagonist which retains its activity following oral doses and has a prolonged duration of action. It is used only in treated opioid addicts as an aid to maintaining their drug-free state.

8

Intramuscular administration of analgesics

The commonest, current practice, on most hospital wards, is to prescribe an analgesic drug on an 'as required' basis. Generally opioid analgesics are administered by the intramuscular route with a dosage interval varying from four to six hours. Many studies have reported the poor quality of analgesia provided by these standard regimes.

Intramuscular administration has gained acceptance because it is relatively simple to perform and does not require nurses with specialist training or medical staff. The 'as required' prescription has achieved popularity for reasons which include the following.

- Fear of overdose — the staff have control over the number of doses administered.
- It is easy to give and requires fewer doses than regular administration.
- Administration occurs as a result of patient demand and therefore the regime is often thought to be optimal.

As a result of widespread use and familiarity with the technique it is generally safe but often ineffective. Although the dose may be sufficient, given intermittently, on an 'as required' basis, by the intramuscular route there can be long periods when the patient will be in pain. This is a result of the lag time between demands for analgesia and the absorption and distribution of the drug after intramuscular injection producing effective analgesia. Even when prescribed four-hourly, most patients will receive only three doses in 24 hours. Furthermore, this regimen can be inflexible; standard doses may not control pain of irregular severity. A rigid regime may not take account of individual variations in analgesic requirements, or variations within the individual patient with time.

The analgesia provided by intermittent intramuscular injections could be improved by:

- more frequent administration;
- regular administration;
- depot preparations of opioids;
- opioids with long duration of action such as buprenorphine.

More frequent administration of analgesics, especially before painful procedures, or regular injections given before the pain has recurred, will benefit the patient. The time during which the patient is in pain will be reduced, and if observations of the patient's general condition and pain control are made before each administration (with appropriate guidelines for withholding doses), then overdosage is unlikely. It should be remembered that acute pain decreases with time and therefore prescriptions for regular opioid administration should have a limited time span (24–36 hours) and be regularly reviewed.

Long-acting opioids may be useful in improving pain control when given intramuscularly. The partial agonist buprenorphine has a duration of analgesia of 6–8 hours after intramuscular injection. It may also be given regularly at six-hourly intervals. Partial agonists are safer when they accumulate than full agonists like morphine whose depressant effects will become dangerous. Methadone also has a prolonged duration of action and this drug may accumulate, if given too frequently, and the interval between doses should be increased with regular administration.

SITES FOR INTRAMUSCULAR INJECTIONS AND THEIR COMPLICATIONS

The commonest sites for administration of intramuscular injections are the buttock and the thigh. In some patients the deltoid region may also be used. Complications of intramuscular injections include the following:

- Bruising when patients have coagulation disturbances or are receiving anticoagulant therapy.
- Damage to the sciatic nerve may occur when injections are made into the butttock. This is the largest nerve in the body

and enters the region of the buttock approximately midway between the ischial tuberosity and the greater trochanter and then travels vertically down the back of the thigh to the popliteal fossa. The safe area for injections into the buttocks is the upper outer quadrant, remembering that the full extent of the buttock region includes the area upwards to the iliac crest and laterally to the greater trochanter.

● Intramuscular injections of opioids are ineffective and dangerous in hypovolaemic patients in whom muscle blood flow is very low. In this group of patients the drugs are poorly absorbed from the muscle bed and hence accumulate. After resuscitation, when muscle blood flow improves, they may experience sudden and unexpected respiratory depression as a result of opioid reabsorption.

In summary, intramuscular opioid administration is generally safe and convenient but provides poor analgesia in some patients in acute pain. Recognition of its failings and improvements in technique may alleviate some of these problems. Regular assessment of the patient is essential to ensure adequate analgesia and maintain patient safety.

9

Opioid infusions

The standard prescription of intermittent analgesic drug regimens commonly leads to inadequate pain control. Improvement may be achieved using some form of continuous analgesic drug administration technique. This may have several advantages including:

- avoidance of troughs in plasma drug concentrations (resulting in pain) which occur with intermittent dosage schedules;
- avoidance of high-peak plasma concentrations (causing adverse effects) after bolus administration.

Continuous intravenous infusions should result in a constant level of analgesia for the duration of the infusion, avoiding periods of inadequate pain relief and periods of excessive sedation from intermittent high concentrations of drug by the administration of repeated bolus doses.

PHARMACOKINETICS OF DRUG ADMINISTRATION

When a continuous intravenous infusion is given, concentrations of drug in the plasma increase slowly with time. At a fixed rate of infusion it will take three to four times the elimination half life of the drug (see page 39) to reach 95 per cent of the steady-state plasma concentration.

A *low* rate of infusion may only attain an effective concentration once it has reached steady state (that is, it will take three to four half lives' duration to become effective as an analgesic).

A *high* rate of infusion will reach effective concentrations more quickly but will equilibrate at a toxic steady-state concentration.

To achieve therapeutic concentrations rapidly it is common to start the infusion at a high rate for a short period of time, then reduce it to one or two lower rates, and then to a final maintenance rate. Alternatively, a loading dose of the drug can be given as a bolus and the infusion started at a maintenance rate (Fig. 9.1).

Attempts have been made to calculate rates of infusion from individual drug pharmacokinetic data and by using computer models, the aim being to produce satisfactory analgesia quickly and without risk of drug accumulation. Studies of the opioid drugs pethidine and alfentanil have produced guidelines for the infusion of these drugs. However, there remain several problems with these techniques.

- There is wide individual variation in the plasma concentrations that give effective analgesia. Calculations designed to

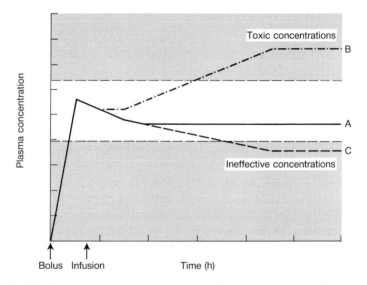

Fig. 9.1 Graph showing plasma concentration plotted against time after initial bolus, for continuous intravenous infusions after the same loading dose of analgesic. Plasma concentrations in the upper shaded area are toxic; those in the lower shaded area are ineffective. Thus curve A shows the ideal infusion rate; curve B shows too high an infusion rate, resulting in accumulation; and curve C shows too low a rate, resulting in ineffective analgesia.

produce a given plasma drug concentration will be ineffective in some patients whilst causing toxicity in others.

- Pharmacokinetically derived infusion rates will still produce widely different plasma drug concentrations in individual patients. In one study using pethidine it was found that the resulting plasma concentrations varied fourfold between patients. Other drugs given to the patient may interfere with the elimination of some of the opioids.

- Increased vigilance is required when the rate of infusion is changed to avoid errors. When the rate requires adjustment several times over a short period there is an increased risk of incorrect rates being set.

SETTING UP OPIOID INFUSIONS

Route of drug administration

The intravenous route is the standard approach. This provides direct access to the circulation and is not dependent upon any variability in drug absorption.

The subcutaneous route is an alternative in those patients requiring analgesia for whom maintenance of IV access is difficult. The technique involves the placement of fine gauge, short intravenous cannulae such as 23 G Y-Can (Wallace) made from Teflon or a winged 23 G needle (Abbott) into the subcutaneous tissues. (Although the Teflon cannulae may kink, they are less likely to produce tissue inflammation.) Positioning the cannula over the chest wall or abdomen can be particularly helpful since at these sites there will be minimal interference with the patient's activities. Appropriate infusion devices for this technique include the small, portable, battery-operated syringe drivers which encourage patient mobility.

When the subcutaneous route is used there may be considerable variability in the rate of drug absorption. Even after stopping the infusion there may be a depot of drug in the subcutaneous tissues to be absorbed. The rate of drug absorption is dependent upon the amount of fat present, which is poorly perfused with blood. Additionally, if the patient develops a low cardiac output the blood flow to the subcutaneous tissues will be further reduced. In such circumstances the analgesic drug will be poorly absorbed and pain will recur, resulting in peripheral vasoconstriction and a further decrease in drug absorption. During this time, drug continues to be deposited and when blood flow improves, toxic amounts of drug may be absorbed. Despite these difficulties this route has been used very successfully.

Choice of drug

Several factors are important in making the decision about which drug should be used.

Familiarity

Whenever opioid infusions are to be prescribed, the doctor and nursing staff who will be monitoring the patient should be familiar with the dosage, effects, and side-effects of the drug prescribed.

Availability

To be suitable for use by infusion the drug chosen should be available in an appropriate formulation. Subcutaneous infusions, for example, will require low-volume infusion rates. Diamorphine is particularly soluble in water and has high potency, therefore high concentrations can be given in a small volume, making it an appropriate choice for this route.

Duration of action

Analgesics with a short duration of action are often recommended for use by infusion. With such drugs there will be a rapid reduction in effect once the infusion is reduced or discontinued, and hence quick recovery from the adverse effects.

Lack of active metabolites

Some drugs have potentially toxic metabolites. For example, the opioid drug pethidine is metabolized to norpethidine in the liver. This metabolite is a central nervous system stimulant and may accumulate when pethidine is given by continuous infusion, producing restlessness and irritability, particularly in patients with some degree of renal failure.

Adverse effects

Prolonged drug administration may be associated with an increased incidence of adverse effects. This may result from accumulation of the drug or of its metabolites. Analgesic agents with a low incidence of adverse effects would therefore be most appropriate for continuous infusion. All opioids will produce some nausea and vomiting and when given by a continuous infusion, antiemetic drugs will need to be regularly administered or even added to the opioid infusion.

When to start an infusion

Patients in severe pain, those whose analgesic requirements are not met by the prescription of regular doses of opioid, and those in intensive care who require frequent doses of analgesic agents may all benefit from a continuous infusion of an analgesic agent.

Suitable opioid drugs and infusion rates are shown in Table 9.1

Table 9.1 Commonly used opioid infusion regimes for adults

Drug	Infusion rates
Morphine	1–5 mg/h
Papaveretum	1–8 mg/h
Pethidine	10–50 mg/h

Requirements

IV access should preferably be through an infusion line used solely for the analgesic drug. If other agents are being administered through the line check their compatibility.

If the syringe pump is to be run with an IV infusion via a Y connector, this should ideally have a one-way valve to prevent the syringe pump emptying into the infusion bag if there is an obstruction at the intravenous cannula.

Patient monitoring

A protocol should be developed with the nursing staff who will care for the patients. This should include the frequency and type of

CONTINUOUS ANALGESIA PUMP		Name –	
Drug :– _____			
For dilution details see prescription chart		Hospital No.	
[Add _____ mg to _____ ml of _____]		Consultant	
		Pain Score (aim at 0 - 1)	
Dilution :– _____ mg/ml		0 = none 1 = slight	
		2 = significant 3 = severe	
Starting rate :– _____ ml/h		**Call MO if:**	
		Pain not controlled	
Range :– _____ to _____ ml/h		Respiratory rate falls below 8	
		Patient not easily rousable	

Date –

Time	Pain Score	Respiration Rate	Pump Setting	Syringe Reading	Initials	Time	Pain Score	Respiration Rate	Pump Setting	Syringe Reading	Initials
1 am						1 am					
2						2					
3						3					
4						4					
5						5					
6 am						6 am					
7						7					
8						8					
9						9					
10						10					
11						11					
Noon						Noon					
1						1					
2						2					
3						3					
4						4					
5						5					
6 pm						6 pm					
7						7					
8						8					
9						9					
10						10					
11						11					
MN						MN					

Fig. 9.2 Hospital chart for monitoring patient with continuous analgesia pump.

Table 9.2 Monitoring patients receiving continuous opioid infusions

The system must be initiated by the anaesthetist concerned.

Aim
To provide safe and reliable analgesia by means of a constant infusion using a syringe pump. Suitable infusions are:
Pethidine   600 mg in 60 ml (i.e. 10 mg/ml)
Morphine   60 mg in 60 ml (i.e. 1 mg/ml)
Average dose required is 2–6 ml per hour

Monitor and record
1. pulse and blood pressure, as indicated surgically
2. pain score, hourly
3. respiration rate, hourly
4. pump setting (ml/h)
5. amount of fluid remaining in syringe, hourly
6. nurse's initials

Aim at:
A pain score of 0–1 and a responsive patient at all times (i.e. a patient may be sleeping but should easily awake and respond to command).

Nursing actions
If patient is still in pain, increase rate by 1 ml/h.
If patient is too sleepy, stop infusion for 1 hour and then restart at new rate 1 ml/h less than previous rate.
Call doctor if:
1. patient is unrousable
2. if pain control is totally inadequate
3. if respiratory rate falls below 8 per min

Medical actions
1. If patient is unrousable, check airway and circulation. Stop infusion of analgesics until condition improves. Consider use of narcotic antagonist e.g. naloxone 0.1 mg IV repeated as necessary.
2. If pain control is totally inadequate, give bolus of analgesic equal to current 1-hour dose and review after 10 min. Consider further bolus injection if pain control still poor. When pain controlled, increase infusion rate by 1 ml/h above previous rate.
3. If respiratory rate is less than 8, stop infusion of narcotics and continue to review hourly until respiration rate is 8 or more. Then start infusion at half the previous rate.

observations, details of drug prescribing, and safety instructions for all patients receiving opioid infusions. A separate chart should be available to facilitate regular recording of infusion rate, dose delivered, and patient observations (notably pulse, blood pressure, respiratory rate, and a simple assessment of the level of analgesia and sedation of the patient).

Guidelines should be agreed as to when to reduce or discontinue the infusion and also to adjustment of infusion rates if analgesia remains inadequate.

Suggested guidelines for the monitoring of patients with opioid infusions are shown in Fig. 9.2 and Table 9.2

DISADVANTAGES WITH CONTINUOUS INFUSIONS OF OPIOIDS

Drug accumulation may occur if the infusion is maintained at an unnecessarily high rate in the face of a changing clinical situation. This will be particularly evident if the patient's ability to eliminate the drug is changing. For example, the development of renal impairment in a patient receiving morphine may reduce the elimination of the active metabolites of morphine, resulting in toxicity.

Infusion rates should be reduced in patients showing signs of impaired cardiovascular function or those who become hypovolaemic, perhaps as a consequence of continued postoperative bleeding. Liver blood flow in these patients may be reduced resulting in a consequent decrease in the rate of drug elimination.

Mechanical failures or the incorrect setting of the equipment can lead to patients receiving too much or too little drug.

Postoperative analgesic requirements vary widely between individuals and within individuals. For example, increased levels of pain will be experienced with movement, physiotherapy, and turning. A fixed-dose infusion may not be flexible enough to provide adequate analgesia in all these instances.

The technique is complex and there is greater risk of prescription and technical errors.

The use of any infusion system requires careful clinical monitoring. The patients must be observed frequently so that the level of infusion can be adjusted to maintain good analgesia with minimum adverse effects.

Nursing staff require additional training to ensure that they are familiar with the equipment and know how to check that it is functioning correctly.

Any equipment at the bedside which is capable of adjustment is open to abuse from the patients themselves or from relatives or visitors who may alter infusion rates. Ideally all infusion systems should have rate controls that are tamper-proof.

ALTERNATIVE METHODS

Pharmaceutical companies have developed drug formulations to provide a slow, controlled release of drug from a depot given orally or applied topically. This endeavours to maintain a steady plasma concentration of drug — similar to those seen with continuous intravenous infusions — throughout a prolonged period. Analgesic preparations that are available include both opioid drugs and some NSAIDs. Oral slow-release preparations include morphine, indomethacin, and diclofenac.

10

Patient-controlled analgesia (PCA) systems

THE BENEFITS OF PCA

The development and introduction of PCA systems into clinical practice has endeavoured to provide a method of analgesia which will bypass any difficulties relating to inappropriate dosing schedules, unpredictable drug absorption, or patient variability. It is a system that also avoids dependence upon the nurses or doctors to provide analgesic medication. These people may be unavailable at times or occupied with other tasks; reliance upon them for analgesia may therefore be a factor in the failure of current regimes to provide satisfactory analgesia. With the PCA systems the patient is in control of their analgesia all the time. Not only does the PCA system provide improved analgesia, it also allows patients to feel in control of their pain.

This technique has been widely practised in midwifery for women in labour, originally with the use of nitrous oxide and air and currently with nitrous oxide in oxygen (Entonox). When PCA is used for opioid administration, a reservoir of drug is maintained and a specifically designed infusion device allows a fixed quantity of drug to be administered in response to patient demand. These systems are most commonly used for the administration of opioid drugs by the intravenous route (which is discussed in this chapter) but they have also been used for epidural and subcutaneous routes of administration.

Safety features of the system include a lock-out interval setting (a time during which the system will not respond to additional patient demands). This can be adjusted to prevent the patient demanding an overdose of analgesic whilst still allowing him or her sufficient analgesic agent to control the pain. Should patients become sedated, their demands for analgesia will reduce, allowing recovery.

The typical pattern of bolus demands made by patients using a PCA system shows a high rate initially (the loading dose), followed by a more stable period of maintenance demands. However, there may be periods of less frequent demands (such as during sleep), followed by periods of catching up with increased demands. Periods of increased demand for improved analgesia may be associated with physiotherapy, mobilization, and other nursing procedures.

SETTING THE PCA PUMP: THE PRESCRIPTION VARIABLES

Since the early development of PCA systems, initially as a research tool and subsequently for clinical use, the equipment has been refined. Various elements of the drug administration regimen can be altered and these are now discussed.

Choice of drug

Experimental studies have shown that PCA systems have been successful with a number of different opioids for relieving acute pain. The most commonly used drug is morphine. Other useful opioids are diamorphine and pethidine.

The ideal analgesic drug for use in PCA systems would have a rapid onset of action with an intermediate duration of action to enhance the control of analgesia. A low incidence of side-effects and a lack of drug interactions would be advantageous. The most widely used opioids in PCA systems are morphine and pethidine. The duration of action of buprenorphine and methadone may be too long for them to gain widespread favour, while fentanyl and its analogues may be too short acting.

Agonist–antagonist opioid drugs exhibit a ceiling effect to their analgesia and respiratory-depressant effects. These drugs may therefore be useful alternatives for use in PCA systems with a reduced risk of respiratory depression.

Size of the bolus dose

This setting allows bolus doses of predetermined size to be delivered. The choice of bolus dose size should be that drug dose which will produce analgesia with low incidence of side-effects. In adults, a bolus dose of 1 mg of morphine is an effective bolus dose. A lower dose produces inadequate analgesia whilst doses of 2 mg are associated, in some patients, with a higher incidence of respiratory depression. PCA systems used in children calculate the bolus dose on body weight.

Bolus dose infusion rate

Most PCA systems allow the bolus dose to be given as a short infusion. This reduces the incidence of side-effects which may be related to high plasma drug concentrations occurring after rapid bolus injections.

Lock-out interval

The lock-out time interval needs to be short enough to allow the patient to administer the drug at high initial rates soon after starting the system, but not so short as to allow overdosage later. The time interval should also take into account the time taken for each bolus dose to prove effective. With too short a time interval, demands may be made before doses previously given have been effective, leading to overdosage. The most commonly used time intervals are of the range 5–10 minutes.

Background infusion rate

The concept of the use of a background infusion at first appears theoretically sound. A background infusion can be used to maintain analgesia with a facility for additional bolus doses available on demand. This may be a useful regimen for drugs with a short duration of action when plasma concentrations may decrease rapidly at times when the patient fails to make demands (for example, while sleeping, when pain relief will be inadequate on awakening). However, doubt remains as to its efficacy. Furthermore, a background infusion may contribute to the development of acute drug tolerance without significantly improving analgesia.

This method has sometimes been referred to as patient-augmented analgesia. Current opinion is against the use of background infusions as they increase the risk of side-effects without improving analgesia. However they are still used in small children when in an ICU, where they are believed to improve sleeping patterns.

Maximum dose rate

Some devices set a maximum dose rate. This may be as a maximum amount of drug per hour or each four-hour period. This is a further safety feature and allows the use of shorter lock-out periods since only a fixed maximum amount of drug for a given time interval is released.

Bolus dose and variable infusion

This setting requires a more complicated, microprocessor-controlled infusion system which can alter the rate of background infusion depending upon the number of patient demands made for bolus doses. For example, a patient with inadequate analgesia will make frequent demands. The device will then set the background infusion at a higher rate. Similarly, it will reduce the rate of the background infusion when the patient is making infrequent demands.

The most commonly used systems in clinical practice are the bolus demand systems with or without the facility for a constant background infusion. Two commonly used PCA systems

Table 10.1 Guidelines for bolus doses and lock-out intervals using opioids in PCA systems

Opioid	Bolus dose (mg)	Lock-out time interval (min)
Morphine	0.5–3	5–20
Pethidine	5–30	5–15
Methadone	0. 5–3	10–20
Nalbuphine	1–5	5–15
Buprenorphine	0.03–0.2	10–20
Hydromorphone	0.1–0.6	5–15
Oxymorphone	0.1–0.6	5–15

in the UK are the Graseby PCAS and the Abbott Lifecare PCAS. Both systems allow for bolus demands with or without a background infusion. They also have variable rates of giving a bolus and this enables them to be administered as a short infusion.

Table 10.1 lists some opioid drugs and doses which have been used in PCA systems to provide analgesia for acute pain.

PATIENT MONITORING

Figure 10.1 gives details of the guidelines in use at Addenbrooke's Hospital, Cambridge, for nursing care of patients using a PCA system. Figure 10.2 is the chart used to record the results of patient monitoring.

With all patients, the monitoring must include an assessment of the pain. Methods and rating scales have been discussed in Chapter 2. Simple methods are useful for continuous assessment and problem patients should be easily identified.

Procedures to be followed in patients with inadequate pain control or those with unwanted or dangerous drug effects must be clearly written on the chart.

In addition, schedules should record the prescribed settings for the PCA system and checks on drug administration to ensure that the equipment is functioning correctly.

HAZARDS ASSOCIATED WITH PCA SYSTEMS

Although patient control of the administration of the drug is a safety feature of the PCA system, there remain hazards through their incorrect use.

Prescription errors

- Inappropriate demand dose.
- Incorrect lock-out interval.
- High background infusion.

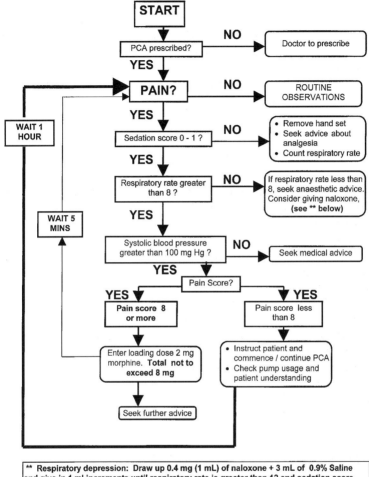

START

PCA prescribed? — **NO** → Doctor to prescribe

YES

PAIN? — **NO** → ROUTINE OBSERVATIONS

YES

Sedation score 0 - 1 ? — **NO** → • Remove hand set • Seek advice about analgesia • Count respiratory rate

YES

Respiratory rate greater than 8 ? — **NO** → If respiratory rate less than 8, seek anaesthetic advice. Consider giving naloxone, **(see ** below)**

YES

Systolic blood pressure greater than 100 mg Hg ? — **NO** → Seek medical advice

YES

Pain Score?

YES → Pain score 8 or more

YES → Pain score less than 8

Enter loading dose 2 mg morphine. **Total not to exceed 8 mg**

• Instruct patient and commence / continue PCA • Check pump usage and patient understanding

Seek further advice

WAIT 1 HOUR

WAIT 5 MINS

** **Respiratory depression: Draw up 0.4 mg (1 mL) of naloxone + 3 mL of 0.9% Saline and give in 1 ml increments until respiratory rate is greater than 12 and sedation score less than 2.**

Ria Sapsford & Sara Kinna C.N.S. Acute Pain, Dept. of Anaesthesia

Fig. 10.1 Guidelines for nursing care of patients using a PCA system.

Provision errors

- Incorrect drug concentration prepared.
- Accidental drug administration. This can occur when new syringes are connected or when partially empty syringes are

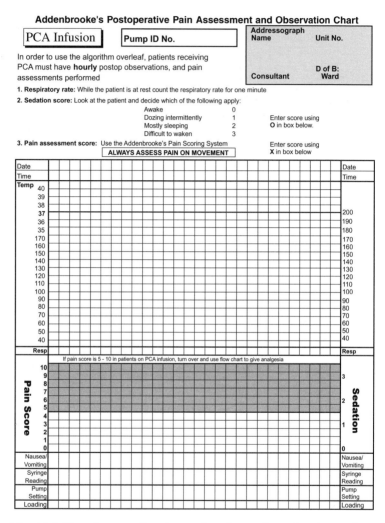

Fig. 10.2 Chart for recording the nursing observations of patients using a PCA system.

removed. The infusion line should be disconnected or cross clamped prior to these manoeuvres.

- Absent or incorrectly placed one-way valves in the infusion system may affect the amount of drug administered, with the analgesic being diverted into reservoir bags of intravenous fluids or other drugs administered through the same intra-venous line.

- Syringes which are not correctly placed within the infusion system can administer excessive drug doses due to siphoning of the drug from the syringe. The Abbott system manu-facturers have developed purpose designed tubing for

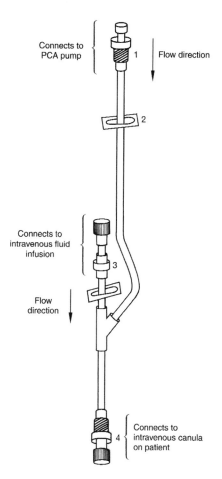

Fig. 10.3 Abbott PCA infusion set (No 3559): (1) anti-siphon valve; (2) slide clamp; (3) back-check valve; (4) secure lock and male adaptor. The presence of valves (1) and (3) prevents fluid entering the PCA pump and the pump emptying into the bag of fluid if there is a blockage at (4).

connecting to their PCA system which includes an anti-siphon device to prevent this occurring (Fig. 10.3).

● Some of the earlier PCA systems (those holding the syringes vertically) have been known to empty spontaneously if placed above the patient. Therefore these should be placed at the level of the patient and not above them.

Patient factors

● Failure to understand the PCA system should not occur because patients should be assessed for their suitability and the system should be properly explained, preoperatively. With most patients, such a problem can be overcome by careful instruction and discussion of the benefits of the system, although there may remain patients who cannot be sufficiently well motivated to use the system.

● Intentional abuse may occur in patients who are generally susceptible to the mood-elevating effects of the opioid analgesics. It does appear to be a very rare hazard.

● People, other than the patient, including relatives, have been known to administer additional boluses to the patient, resulting in excessive sedation.

Equipment malfunction

Excess or inadequate drug administration may occur with equipment failure. Syringes may empty at faster or slower rates than programmed if incorrect sizes or specifications of syringes are used in individual PCA systems.

INADEQUATE ANALGESIA WITH PCA SYSTEMS

When the degree of pain relief patients obtain using PCA systems is assessed, it is noteworthy that often patients do not administer sufficient analgesia to completely abolish their pain despite the ability to do so. The reasons for this are complex. Patients may not envisage complete analgesia as being possible, or there may be failure to understand the system or fear of the adverse effects of the drugs administered. In addition, staff may encourage caution, discouraging patients from making demands unless really necessary or to 'be careful not to use too much'.

Even when all of these difficulties have been excluded, patients still do not relieve their pain completely. It may be that a small amount of pain, sufficient to cause discomfort, but not distress, is necessary to protect the patient from harm. Alternatively, a minor degree of discomfort may be preferable to the unwanted effects of the drug.

Inadequate analgesia may also result from practical errors in the use of the PCA system, including the following.

Incorrect prescriptions

A prescription for too small or infrequent doses of the analgesic drug is an obvious cause of failure. In addition, unnecessarily large doses may be prescribed, leading to unpleasant side-effects — as a consequence the patient may prefer to suffer the pain rather than the adverse effects of the drug.

Equipment failure

Problems with the pump or its connections can result in excessive or reduced drug administration. Connections of the equipment should be routinely checked and the levels of drug remaining in the reservoir or syringe recorded, allowing a further check on the amount of drug that the machine has delivered.

Shared intravenous access

PCA systems should not share intravenous access sites with other infusion lines without a one-way valve being incorporated into each solution-delivery set. If the PCA system is connected to an intravenous access site without a one-way valve it is possible for the pump to direct the analgesic agent into the tubing and reservoir of the IV bag. This will result in inadequate analgesia with an additional risk of the drug being administered in a large bolus from the other IV infusion if this is then given quickly.

Psychological factors

The degree of pain tolerated by patients will vary enormously depending upon psychological and social factors. In addition, the patient's personality and other psychological factors may be a reason for the patient aiming at a tolerable level of pain rather than complete analgesia; he or she may believe that a need to suffer is part of the healing process.

USES OF PCA SYSTEMS

Clinical

Postoperative pain

PCA systems are being increasingly used in hospitals for the management of postoperative pain. They are principally used for patients undergoing major surgery, although increased availability of the equipment may allow their wider use.

Obstetrics

The technique was first used to provide analgesia for women in labour using nitrous oxide — originally in air and now in oxygen. Intravenous opioids are now used both in labour and to provide postoperative analgesia following Caesarean section deliveries.

Trauma

The PCA system offers the advantage of good pain control with avoidance of excessive sedation.

Burns

Patients require analgesia not only for their thermal injury but will also experience increased requirements for pain control during procedures such as wound cleaning and changes of dressing. Standard methods of analgesic administration would allow additional bolus doses to be given before these procedures. However, patients will vary in the amount of drug required — not only between individuals, but also in the same patient at different times during recovery. Even using this regime, patients will still not receive sufficient analgesia for these procedures. Therefore allowing patients access to a PCA system will enable self-administration of analgesia to levels which give comfort during the procedures.

Paediatrics

The use of PCA systems for children has been rising, limited by the age of a child who can understand what they need to do to receive analgesia. This usually means that the child must be 5–6 years of age. If analgesia is inadequate it is safer to reduce the lock-out interval rather than increase the bolus. A background infusion in small children is helpful in improving the child's sleeping pattern especially in the first 24–48 hours after an operation.

More recently there has been a trend towards the use of parent- and patient-controlled analgesia or parent-assisted analgesia. In this situation the parent, who is staying in the same room as the child, is also instructed in the use of the PCA system and may make demands to improve the pain control as well as the child. In early reports most parents have found this useful, although others have expressed anxiety about being in charge of the system. Nurse-controlled analgesia (NCA) is another variant of this technique.

The dosing guidelines used at Addenbrooke's Hospital, Cambridge, for use of PCA and NCA opioids in children are shown in Tables 10.2 and 10.3. The guidelines for care of children on PCA systems are given in Fig. 10.4.

Terminal care

PCA systems can be used in hospital for the management of acute exacerbation of the patient's pain or worsening of the clinical condition. They are also finding use in ambulatory patients — a

Table 10.2 How to make up infusions used in PCA for children

Technique	Standard infusions	Maximum 4-hrly dose
Weight up to 40 Kg (PCA)	Morphine sulphate 0.5 mg/kg in 50 ml 0.9% saline gives 10 µg/kg/ml	400 µg/kg
Weight >40 Kg (PCA)	Morphine sulphate 1.0 mg/kg in 50 ml 0.9% saline gives 20 µg/kg/ml	400 µg/kg
NCA	Morphine sulphate 0.5 mg/kg in 50 ml 0.9% saline gives 10 µg/kg/ml	400 µg/kg

Table 10.3 How to program PCA pumps for use with children

Circumstances	Loading dose (μg/kg)	Background infusion (μg/kg/h)	Bolus dose	Lock-out time (min)
PCA in patient up to 40 kg	50–100	4	10–20 μg/kg	5–15
PCA in patient >40 kg	50–100	0	1–2 mg	5–15
NCA	50–100	0–20	10–20 μg/kg	20–60
NCA in intensive care	50–100	0–20	10–20 μg/kg	5–10

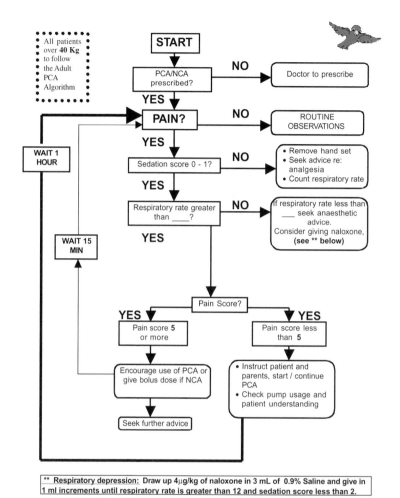

Fig. 10.4 Guidelines for nursing care of children using a PCA system.

particular benefit being the ability to administer epidural opioids by the PCA apparatus, for longer-term pain control.

Research

PCA systems are widely used in the assessment of new analgesic agents. In the management of acute pain, patients can be given the new analgesic drug or a placebo while also allowing them access to a PCA system with a conventional opioid such as morphine, to provide analgesia on demand. The efficacy of the new agent can then be compared with the placebo effect by looking at the reductions in the amount of morphine required to provide analgesia in the two groups, the so-called 'morphine sparing' effect.

Similarly it can be used to compare the efficacy of preoperative psychological preparation in improving postoperative analgesia by comparing morphine requirements in the different groups.

COMMON SIDE-EFFECTS

Nausea and vomiting

The incidence of nausea whilst on PCA has been estimated to be around 60 per cent, whilst for vomiting, the estimates vary between 30–40 per cent. Prophylactic antiemetics and the administration of an antiemetic with the PCA opioid could combat this problem. Both of these areas require further research as there have been conflicting reports showing benefit and no benefit. Droperidol added to the PCA opioid has been shown in many studies to reduce the incidence of nausea and vomiting as well as the need for rescue antiemetics. However it has also caused increased sedation.

Respiratory depression

There have been no significant differences in the incidence of respiratory depression between patients receiving conventional pain management and those receiving PCA. For a given level of effective analgesia, there is less risk of respiratory depression with PCA than other methods of opioid administration. This may be because PCA minimizes fluctuations in blood levels of opioids and allows the patient to titrate opioid requirements to the level of pain experienced.

Respiratory depression may occur if:

- people other than the patient activate the PCA system;
- a background infusion is used;
- technical faults result in fast infusions of high opioid doses;

- a IV catheter becomes extravascular (tissuing) and a sub-cutaneous depot builds up;
- the prescription is inappropriate.

DISADVANTAGES OF PCA SYSTEMS

Cost

The initial cost of equipment for this technique is high. At present, PCA systems cost between £2000 to £4000. To provide these systems for every patient in acute pain who may benefit would require a large capital outlay. Evidence of cost saving as a result of using PCA systems can only be envisaged in terms of a reduction in nursing time spent in duties relating to the provision of analgesia for the patients, allowing more time for other patient needs. Improvement in analgesia may also produce the benefits of reduced morbidity and length of hospital stay, and thereby provide cost savings.

Monitoring

Although these systems have an inherent safety feature in that the patients themselves make the demands, it is easy to overestimate the safety and become complacent. The use of these techniques does not obviate the need for close monitoring of the patients or vigilance in observing side-effects of the drugs used. Reports of both nursing staff and relatives administering unnecessary analgesic drug boluses for patients may be few, but they indicate that the present systems must be monitored.

11

Inflammation and non-steroidal anti-inflammatory drugs

INTRODUCTION

Though the initial pain of injury is due to traumatic activation of nociceptors, the persistence of pain at the site of injury is caused by inflammatory mediators released by damaged tissue as well as increased spinal cord sensitivity to nerve impulses from the damaged area.

Peripheral mechanisms of inflammatory pain revolve around the localized sensitization of nociceptors by prostaglandins and leukotrienes. These prostaglandins and leukotrienes increase the pain response to other chemical mediators such as histamine and bradykinin, which are released in response to cell damage from trauma. The characteristic signs of inflammation are described as 'rubor, dolor, and tumor' — erythema, pain, and swelling — and result from the effects of these mediators on peripheral vessels. These substances produce vasodilatation (rubor), nociception (resulting in pain), and increased capillary permeability (resulting in swelling).

The analgesic and anti-inflammatory properties of some plant extracts (now recognized as containing salicylates) have been known from earliest times. Records of their uses have been found in Egyptian papyri and they were widely used in early Roman and Greek medicine.

The nineteenth century saw the preparation of salicylic acid, initially from natural sources and later from chemical synthesis. The preparation of aspirin (acetyl salicylic acid) was reported in 1853 by Charles Gerhardt, Professor of Chemistry in Strasbourg, but its full commercial exploitation did not occur for some 40 years. Early investigators using salicylates recognized the gastric irritant effects and also that this could be relieved by the administration of sodium bicarbonate. High doses of salicylates were employed therapeutically in the management of acute rheumatic illnesses. Nausea, vomiting, and tinnitus, due to toxicity, were common side-effects. The early physician's therapeutic indications for these agents recognized their analgesic, antipyretic, and anti-inflammatory effects. These features are still important today.

Salicylates are probably the most well recognized of drugs that now fall into the category of mild analgesics with anti-inflammatory activity classed as non-steroidal anti-inflammatory agents (NSAIDs).

MECHANISM OF ACTION OF NSAIDS

Generally all agents will have analgesic effects but there may be considerable variations in their anti-inflammatory activity (for example, indomethacin has potent anti-inflammatory effects, whereas paracetamol has none). These agents predominantly act peripherally at the site of injury rather than in the central nervous system where opioid drugs principally act. They inhibit cyclo-oxygenase dependent prostaglandin synthesis.

Two forms of cyclo-oxygenase, COX1 and COX2, have been identified. COX1 is a normal constituent of cells and is involved in producing the prostaglandins regulating functions like renal blood flow and gastric mucus production. COX2 is induced in response to tissue damage and produces the prostaglandins causing sensitization of nociceptors. Thus research is being directed to produce COX2-selective inhibitors on the grounds that common side-effects of NSAIDs due to unselected inhibition of COX1 and 2 can be avoided.

Some actions of NSAIDs (for example, antipyretic) may result from prostaglandin inhibition within the central nervous system. Prostaglandins are released in almost all forms of tissue damage and are thought to sensitize the pain receptors to different stimuli such as chemical mediators, heat, and mechanical stimuli. Chemical mediators released during the inflammatory process will interact and produce pain at lower concentrations as a result of this prior sensitization (see Fig. 11.1).

When used as analgesics these agents all exhibit a ceiling effect (a dose beyond which further improvements in analgesia will not

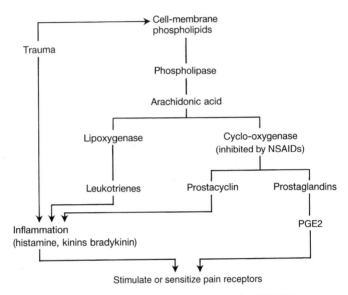

Fig. 11.1 Mechanism of prostaglandin inhibition by NSAIDs.

occur). They are also less likely to produce sedation, respiratory depression, or mood changes.

They are widely used in the control of minor or moderate pain such as headache, toothache, and low back pain for example. When used for musculoskeletal disorders both their analgesic and anti-inflammatory actions are useful. For postoperative pain they have been found to be particularly useful after dental surgery, for example after extraction of wisdom teeth, and parenteral preparations have also been used to provide analgesia after some orthopaedic operations, such as hip replacement. It is thought that their administration preoperatively would inhibit prostaglandin synthesis prior to the tissue disruption of surgery and thereby reduce the requirement for postoperative analgesia, but this remains speculative.

ADVERSE EFFECTS

The following are the most common adverse effects and are summarised in Fig. 11.2. The incidence of adverse drug reactions with the various NSAIDs is listed in Table 11.1

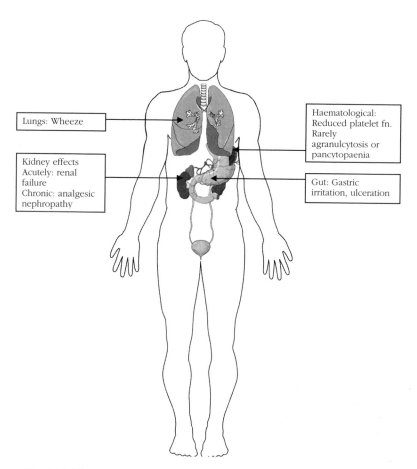

Fig. 11.2 The adverse effects of NSAIDs.

Gastrointestinal effects

These are the most frequently reported side-effects of NSAIDs. Gastric irritation, dyspepsia, and ulceration, often leading to upper-gastrointestinal haemorrhage, have occurred. To reduce the incidence of these problems they can be prescribed in combination with H_2-receptor blocking drugs (cimetidine). Diarrhoea and constipation have also been reported.

Table 11.1 Prescription-related reports of serious gastrointestinal (GI) and other serious reactions (liver, kidney, skin, blood) to some non-steroidal anti-inflammatory drugs during their first five years of marketing

NSAID	Number of prescriptions (millions)	Serious GI reactions per million prescriptions	Other serious reactions per million prescriptions
Azaprapazone	0.91	67.0	20.9
Piroxicam	9.16	58.7	9.4
Naproxen	4.67	32.8	8.4
Diclofenac	3.25	20.9	18.5
Flurbiprofen	3.35	27.4	8.4
Indomethacin SR (withdrawn)	0.44	386.4	18.2
Ketoprofen	3.19	33.2	5.3
Ibuprofen	5.47	6.6	6.6

(Reproduced with permission from: CSM Update, *BMJ* **292**: 1190–1)

Haematological effects

These agents reduce platelet aggregation. This reduction in platelet 'stickiness' has been used therapeutically in the prevention of cerebrovascular accidents and myocardial infarction using low-dose aspirin. Bone marrow suppression, with agranulocytosis, pancytopaenia, and aplastic anaemia have occurred with several different agents.

Renal tract

Combinations of aspirin and phenacetin were well-recognized causes of renal failure — the so-called 'analgesic nephropathy'. Interstitial nephritis as a cause of impaired renal function has also been associated with modern NSAID therapy. Patients at particular risk of renal damage are those who may have impaired renal function or reduced renal perfusion, such as patients with cardiac failure, shock, or patients requiring intensive care.

Fluid balance

These agents produce sodium and water retention, which may lead to cardiac failure in patients with poor myocardial function. They reduce renal blood flow and lead to a reduction in urine production.

Hypersensitivity

Acute bronchospasm, urticaria, and oedema can occur following ingestion of NSAIDs in sensitive patients. This was first recognized with aspirin. These patients generally have a history of asthma and frequently have nasal polyps. Ten per cent of asthmatics are found to be sensitive to NSAIDs. A previous history of safe use of aspirin or ibuprofen without triggering an asthma attack reliably excludes sensitive patients for clinical purposes.

Idiosyncratic reactions

Other more unusual reactions to these agents can occur, including rashes and photosensitivity.

CHOICE OF NSAIDS

Though there are numerous NSAIDs available, no single drug has been shown to be better than the others for its analgesic properties. Meta-analyses which pool the results of several studies to see if any particular NSAID is better than any other for osteoarthritic pain of the hip and knee have not shown any conclusive benefit favouring a particular drug. These studies were limited by a number of factors including different definitions of osteoarthritis and different outcomes measured for analgesia.

Examples of agents from differing chemical classes are now described. For individual drug dosages see Table 11.2

Aspirin (salicylate)

Originally the drug of first choice for mild pain, headache, musculo-skeletal, or arthritic pain. More modern NSAIDs may now be used for some indications as they may be better tolerated. Aspirin is contraindicated in children under 12 years because of its links with Reye's syndrome (a severe illness with high mortality from coma and hepatic failure) except for specific clinical conditions such as juvenile arthritis. There is little anti-inflammatory activity, in adults, with doses less than 3 g daily.

Aspirin has been marketed in numerous formulations in attempts to reduce the gastrointestinal side-effect, which remains the most common reason for stopping treatment.

Indomethacin (cyclic acetic acid)

This drug may be used for pain and moderate to severe inflammation in acute musculoskeletal disorders, and is particularly useful in acute gout. However, its use is associated with a high incidence of adverse effects, notably dizziness, headaches, and gastrointestinal disturbances. Slow-release formulations and suppositories are available and oral doses should be taken with food.

Diclofenac (aryl acetic acids)

This drug is available as an oral sustained-release preparation, as suppository, and also as a parenteral preparation for intramuscular

Table 11.2 Doses of commonly used NSAIDs

Drug	Usual total daily dose (mg)	Usual single dose (mg)	Usual dose interval (h)	Time to peak effect (h)
Aspirin	1800–1600	300–600	4	0.25
Diclofenac	75–150	75	8	1–3
Ibuprofen	1200–2400	300–600	6–8	0.5–1.5
Indomethacin	150–200	25–50	6–12	1–2
Ketoprofen	100–200	25–50	6–8	0.5–2
Ketorolac	40–90	10–30	4–6	0.17–0.5
Naproxen	500–1000	250–500	6–8	1–2
Paracetamol	2000–4000	500–1000	4	1
Phenylbutazone	300–400	100	6–8	2
Piroxicam	20–30	10–20	12–24	2

and intravenous administration. In its parenteral form it is suitable for the relief of pain from renal colic where it has been shown be as effective as other analgesics (see the suggested reading list) or for postoperative pain on its own or in addition to opioids.

Ketorolac (acetic acid derivative)

This NSAID was the first one available for intravenous administration. Oral ketorolac provides analgesia that is the same or better than aspirin, acetaminophen, or dextropropoxyphene with acetaminophen and equal analgesia to ibuprofen and acetaminophen/ codeine preparations. Intramuscular and intravenous ketorolac provides analgesia equivalent to pethidine and morphine.

Its use has been limited by the prolonged onset of analgesic action (30–60 minutes) and by a significant number of patients (around 25 per cent) who exhibit little or no response to it. The incidence of adverse events such as gastrointestinal bleeding, acute renal failure, and bleeding tendencies have decreased since revision of dosage guidelines and by restricting its use to less than 5 days. The suggested dosage for intramuscular or intravenous use (maximum duration 2 days) is an initial bolus of 10 mg followed by 10–30 mg every 4–6 hours with a maximum of 90 mg daily.

Ibuprofen (proprionic acid derivatives)

This is the most widely used agent of this group. As an oral preparation, it is used in mild pain of musculoskeletal type. It has a lower incidence of side-effects compared with other NSAIDs but it has only weak anti-inflammatory action. Other agents in this group include naproxen (an effective anti-inflammatory), fenoprofen, and ketoprofen.

Mefenamic acid (fenamates)

This drug is related to indomethacin and is useful in mild to moderate pain. It has little anti-inflammatory effect and should be administered after food.

Piroxicam (oxicams)

This drug has the benefit of good efficacy with a prolonged duration of action allowing a once-daily dosage schedule. It has a greater incidence of adverse effects than ibuprofen, particularly in the elderly.

Paracetamol (p-amino phenols)

This drug is unusual among the NSAIDs as its action is generally believed to result from the inhibition of prostaglandin production within the central nervous system. It is the most commonly used analgesic agent and is first-line agent for the management of mild and moderate pain. It has replaced aspirin as the analgesic and antipyretic agent of choice in children.

It is usually administered orally although suppository preparations are available. Gastrointestinal side-effects are minimal and the risks of renal and hepatic damage are limited to overdose. Unlike other NSAIDs listed here, paracetamol has almost no anti-inflammatory activity.

Doses:

Adults	0.5–1 g orally, 4–6 hourly
	0.5–1 g suppository, 4–6 hourly
Children	10–15 mg/kg orally, 4–6 hourly
	15–20 mg/kg suppository, 4–6 hourly

SUMMARY: NSAIDS AND ACUTE PAIN

NSAIDs are useful in mild to moderate pain and can be used in combination with opioids for severe pain. They have been proven to reduce the amount of opioid needed for analgesia in severe pain. Nearly all have analgesic effects though their anti-inflammatory effects vary greatly. No evidence exists to show that one NSAID is better than the others for *analgesic* effect.

When prescribing NSAIDs, patients at high risk for common side-effects must be excluded. These include patients giving a history of gastrointestinal ulcers, bleeding problems, or those at high risk of renal failure (pre-existing renal dysfunction, hypo-volaemia). NSAIDs can be useful in postoperative analgesia where the risks can be minimized by careful patient selection and limiting the duration of use to the first 1–3 days after surgery.

12

Pharmacology of local anaesthetic agents

Local anaesthetic agents produce a transient inhibition of nerve impulse conduction. Normally when a nerve transmits an impulse its permeability to sodium is increased, resulting in a change in the electrical state of the cell (depolarization). When local anaesthetics are used the permeability of the cell membrane to sodium is reduced. This results in a slow rate of rise of the depolarization potential and failure to achieve the critical threshold for the propagation of the electrical change (action potential). Local anaesthetics can be used to block the transmission of painful stimuli at any point from the peripheral nerve to the spinal cord.

The basic chemical structures of the local anaesthetic agents in current use are shown in Fig. 12.1.

The local-anaesthetic molecule includes an aromatic and an amine terminal with intermediate chain. They are generally classified according to the chemical nature of the linkage group between the aromatic portion and the intermediate chain structure of the molecule. This group may be an amide or an ester. Amide-linked anaesthetics are generally more stable and are metabolized in the liver. Ester-linked agents are hydrolysed in the plasma.

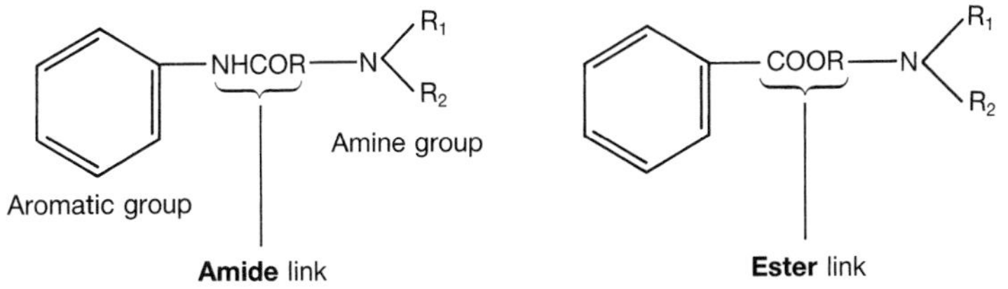

Fig. 12.1 Chemical structure of local anaesthetic agents.

Changes in the chemical structure of the molecules alter the physicochemical properties of the local anaesthetic agent and change the profile of the local anaesthetic activity.

Local anaesthetic agents are weak bases. At the pH of tissues the agents exist in both unionized and ionized forms. Only the unionized form which is lipid soluble will be able to penetrate the cell membranes. The degree of lipid solubility of the agent is therefore important in determining drug potency. The local anaesthetic base is relatively insoluble in water and so is generally prepared as the hydrochloride salt or as the carbonate form, the latter having a more rapid onset. Examples of commonly used local anaesthetic agents are listed in Table 12.1.

Table 12.1 Commonly used local anaesthetic agents

Local anaesthetic	Chemical structure
Lignocaine	Amide
Bupivacaine	Amide
Ropivacaine	Amide
Prilocaine	Amide
Procaine	Ester
Amethocaine	Ester

INDIVIDUAL LOCAL ANAESTHETIC AGENTS

Lignocaine

Lignocaine has become the most widely used local anaesthetic agent. It has good powers of penetration and can be used topically, for infiltration as well as for regional blocks in appropriate concentrations. In addition, by virtue of its membrane-stabilizing effects, it has proved successful in the treatment of ventricular dysrhythmias.

Prilocaine

Prilocaine is more slowly absorbed than lignocaine and so is less dependent upon the addition of vasoconstrictor agents. It has a lower acute toxicity on the central nervous system and is rapidly metabolized in the liver. Side-effects include the development of methaemoglobinaemia after high doses of the drug, which should be treated with intravenous injection of methylene blue (2 mg/kg).

Bupivacaine and L bupivacaine

Bupivacaine is a more potent local anaesthetic drug and has similarly increased toxicity. It has a prolonged duration of local anaesthetic action. The addition of adrenaline (epinephrine) as a vasoconstrictor has minimal effects on the duration of action or toxicity. L or levobupivacaine (also known as S(-)bupivacaine) is currently undergoing clinical evaluation.

Cocaine

This was one of the earliest local anaesthetic agents but is now rarely used therapeutically. It is an effective surface local anaesthetic with marked vasoconstrictor properties, but has now been superseded by less toxic drugs. It is still used in oto-laryngology (ENT surgery) to produce topical local anaesthesia in the nasal airways where its vasoconstrictor effects will reduce bleeding at operation. For topical analgesia in other areas, toxic effects including central nervous system stimulation with excitation, tachycardia, and hypertension preclude its use.

Ropivacaine

Ropivacaine is an amide local anaesthetic introduced into clinical practice in 1996. It arose from research into different biological properties of optical isomers of drugs after case reports of death from bupivacaine toxicity in the early 1980s. Bupivacaine is a racemic mixture of R and S enantiomers and ropivacaine is the purified S enantiomer of a derivative of bupivacaine which has been found to be less cardiotoxic. The toxic dose for ropivacaine is 7.5 mg/kg compared to 2 mg/kg for bupivacaine.

Though the sensory block produced is similar to an equivalent dose of bupivacaine, the motor block is slower in onset, less intense, and of shorter duration. Thus it has been advocated for epidural analgesia in labour and other ambulatory regional anaes-thetic techniques.

EMLA and ametop creams

EMLA stands for 'eutectic mixture of local anaesthetic'. Eutectic means that the constituents (prilocaine and lignocaine) are mixed in such a proportion that the resulting mixture has the lowest melting point possible. In practice, the equally proportioned lignocaine/prilocaine mixture has a melting point of 16°C and thus exists as an oil at room temperature.

Amethocaine has been introduced as ametop gel for topical analgesia. Though its properties as a local anaesthetic have been known for many years, its benefits as a faster acting agent than EMLA have only recently been realized. Neither should be used on burned skin. The two topical agents are compared in Table 12.2.

Dosage guidelines

Fixed maximum doses of local anaesthetic agents can only be a guideline. Sensitivity to any dose will depend upon the size of the patient, site of injection, and presence of vasoconstrictor agents. The addition of vasoconstrictor drugs will generally reduce sensitivity to local anaesthetic agents in all sites of use, except when used topically to the tracheo-bronchial tree where absorption is particularly rapid.

Effective concentrations and volumes of local anaesthetic agent vary widely with the differing techniques. When lignocaine is used, satisfactory infiltration analgesia can be obtained at low concentrations (0.5 per cent) whilst effective motor block during epidural anaesthesia will require higher concentrations (1.5–2 per cent).

The time to onset and duration of effect of commonly used local anaesthetics are listed in Table 12.3.

Absorption of the local anaesthetic agent from the site of injection into tissues and blood vessels is also dependent upon the lipid solubility of the individual agent. As local anaesthetic agents are relatively lipid soluble, diffusion across capillary endothelium will be rapid and systemic absorption rates will be dependent upon blood flow and binding to local tissues. The vascularity of the site of injection is therefore important; rapid and extensive absorption will take place from inflamed and highly vascular tissues.

Table 12.2 A comparison of amethocaine gel (ametop) and EMLA cream

	Age group for use	Onset	Duration of analgesia	Effects
Ametop gel	Not for pre-term babies Not for infants under 1/12	45 min	4–6 h	Vasodilator
EMLA cream	Not under 1 year of age	60–90 min	1 h	Vasoconstrictor

Table 12.3 Time course of actions of local anaesthetic agents and suggested maximum doses

Agent	Onset (min)	Duration (h)	Max dosage (mg/kg)
Lignocaine	10–15	1–3	3
Lignocaine and adrenaline	10–15	3–4	7
Prilocaine	10–15	1.5–2	5
Prilocaine and adrenaline	10–15	2–3	8
Bupivacaine 0.25%	15–30	3–5	2
Bupivacaine 0.5%	15–30	3–6	2
Bupivacaine 0.5% and adrenaline	15–30	3–6	2
Ropivacaine 0.75%	10–20	3–6	7
Ropivacaine 0.75% and adrenaline	10–20	3–6	7

Table 12.4 Absorption of local anaesthetic drugs and site of injection

Site	Absorption
Intercostal	Rapid
Caudal	
Epidural	↕
Brachial plexus	
Sciatic and femoral	Slow

Vasoconstrictor drugs will reduce the vascular absorption of the local anaesthetic agents. In general, systemic absorption rate is related to the site of injection (see Table 12.4). Absorption decreases in the following order:

intercostal>caudal>epidural>brachial plexus>sciatic and *femoral blocks.*

Vasoconstrictor agents such as adrenaline (epinephrine), at concentrations of 1:100 000–1:400 000, as well as phenylephrine, felypressin, and octapressin are often used to reduce drug absorption and prolong the duration of anaesthetic effects. They produce little prolongation of action with the long-acting local anaesthetic agents such as bupivacaine.

TOXICITY OF LOCAL ANAESTHETICS

When administered in an appropriate dose and in a correct anatomical location, local anaesthetics are relatively free from toxic effects. However, local and systemic toxic effects may follow the administration of an excessive dose of local anaesthetic agent or following accidental intravascular or intrathecal injection.

Local effects

Local tissue toxicity

Nerve damage in experimental animals has been seen following excessive doses of local anaesthetic agents. In addition, preservative agents, notably sodium bisulphite, may be neurotoxic. Skeletal muscle changes have been observed with most of the local anaesthetic agents and the irritant properties of local anaesthetic agents may be responsible, although the changes have not correlated with clinically overt signs of local irritation. The damage is reversible and regeneration complete within two weeks.

These effects are mostly experimental and do not appear to cause problems in clinical practice.

Vascular damage

If vasoconstrictor drugs such as adrenaline (epinephrine) are used, spasm of blood vessels may result. In areas of the body supplied by end-arteries (ear lobes, nose, digits, penis) this may result in necrosis. Avoid adrenaline (epinephrine) in these areas.

Systemic effects

Cardiovascular system

Local anaesthetic agents, by virtue of their membrane-stabilizing properties, reduce cardiac irritability, and impulse conduction time is prolonged. All agents are negative inotropes and reduce myocardial contractility. These properties can produce direct impairment of cardiac function if large amounts are absorbed or after inadvertent intravenous injection.

Vasodilatation occurs as a result of direct relaxant effects on smooth muscle with some local anaesthetic agents. In addition, the reduced cardiac output, resulting from the direct cardiac depressant effects, and the hypotension result in tissue hypoxia and a metabolic acidosis. This further impairs myocardial function. Cardiovascular depression resulting from toxic effects of bupivacaine has proved refractory to resuscitation attempts.

An adequate circulation must be established to enable drug redistribution and metabolism of the drug in the liver, and thereby reduce toxic plasma concentrations of bupivacaine. Prolonged cardiopulmonary resuscitation may be required and, on occasions, cardiopulmonary bypass has been instituted to support the cardiovascular system.

Central nervous system

Initially, central nervous system excitation is seen as a result of inhibition of cortical inhibitory synapses, and convulsions will occur. Larger doses will produce generalized central nervous system depression.

Symptoms of toxicity

At the onset of toxic effects, the patient may complain of a feeling of numbness, characteristically of tongue and lips, and general light headedness. Tinnitus and visual disturbance are other frequent complaints that should alert one to the risk of systemic toxicity. Symptoms of toxicity can be summarized as:

- tinnitus
- restlessness
- muscle twitching
- loss of consciousness
- generalized convulsions
- respiratory arrest
- hypotension
- asystole (bupivacaine may produce ventricular dysrhythmias)

Management of systemic toxicity

Drugs and equipment necessary for the management of systemic toxicity of local anaesthetic agents should be available wherever these drugs are used other than for skin infiltration and distal limb nerve blocks, and the operator must be familiar with the treatment required.

Problems may arise as a result of the profound cardiovascular depression which occurs with hypotension and cardiac arrest. The depression of the central nervous system, leading to respiratory depression, hypoxia, and acidosis, may be the primary cause of the collapse, with the cardiovascular problems secondary events. Resuscitation should be directed to improving both of these.

Minimum resuscitation facilities

1. Fully trained staff familiar with cardiopulmonary resuscitation at basic and advanced levels must be available.
2. Oxygen supply, masks, and a self-inflating bag to enable manual assistance of ventilation during resuscitation.
3. Suction apparatus — when consciousness is impaired or lost the patient is at risk of aspiration of gastric contents.
4. Tracheal intubation equipment will be necessary, both to protect the airway in the unconscious patient and for assistance of ventilation. Laryngoscopes and cuffed tracheal tubes of appropriate adult and paediatric sizes should be available.
5. Anticonvulsant drugs should be available — benzodiazepines (for example, diazemuls) or a barbiturate such as thiopentone. Suxamethonium, a short-acting, depolarizing muscle relaxant, may be used by an anaesthetist to facilitate tracheal intubation.
6. Sympathomimetic drugs to treat hypotension may be required. Ephedrine in 5 mg boluses, given intravenously, is effective.
7. Anti-arrhythmic drugs may be necessary. Bradycardia may be treated with intravenous atropine. Adrenaline (epinephrine) will be required in cases of asystole. Other dysrhythmias may improve once hypoxia has been corrected and cardiac output has improved with the previous measures.
8. When performing major conduction nerve blocks such as epidural or spinal blocks, a tilting bed, table, or trolley on which the patient may be rapidly placed in the head down (Trendelenberg) position is essential. This will increase

venous return and, in patients with profound sympathetic blockade after spinal or epidural block, this will counteract the venous pooling in the lower limbs.

Reactions to vasoconstrictor drugs

Vasoconstrictor drugs are used in combination with local anaesthetic agents to retard drug absorption and reduce systemic drug toxicity. In addition, by maintaining effective tissue drug concentrations they prolong the duration of action of some local anaesthetic drugs. Reactions to the vasoconstrictor agent may be seen and are usually related to systemic absorption or intravenous injection. Symptoms include anxiety and palpitations; the patient will appear pale and develop a tachycardia, hypertension, and rapid respiratory rate. These effects are usually transient, the agents being rapidly metabolized.

Allergic reactions to local anaesthetic drugs

These are rare reactions, particularly with the amide group of drugs. When ester drugs such as procaine were commonly used, skin reactions resulting from handling were observed.

Treatment of allergic reactions include general supportive measures to ensure adequate oxygenation and specific therapies to minimize the immunological reactions. Hypotension should initially be managed with intravenous fluids and bronchospasm requires the administration of β_2-adrenoceptor stimulants, the drug of first choice being adrenaline (epinephrine). Steroids may be given intravenously and systemic antihistamines may be administered.

Applications of local analgesic techniques in acute pain

This section provides a brief review of some of the techniques available to relieve acute pain. Some techniques (indicated in the text by an asterisk *) should only be performed by persons trained in anaesthesia.

Topical

Local anaesthetic agents may be applied to mucous membranes to produce localized areas of analgesia. This may be particularly useful in painful lesions of the mouth and oropharynx. Suitable agents include lozenges of benzocaine or amethocaine. A topical, 0.5 per cent solution of amethocaine is available and provides useful anaesthesia of the cornea for procedures such as removal of a foreign body or for analgesia after corneal abrasions.

Topical application of bupivacaine to the donor sites of skin grafts gives good analgesia postoperatively. EMLA cream may also be useful in this situation.

Local infiltration

This method of producing local anaesthesia may be useful after trauma, for example before suturing of simple wounds or for the infiltration of fracture sites prior to manipulation.

Local anaesthetic agents may be infiltrated into surgical wounds at the end of an operation to provide analgesia well into the postoperative period. This is particularly useful after procedures such as orchidopexy and herniotomy in children. Catheters inserted in surgical wounds at the time of operation have also been used to enable intermittent injections of local anaesthetic agents to be repeated in the postoperative period to provide prolonged analgesia. However, the analgesia produced is often patchy and concern that the presence of the catheter in the wound may increase the risk of postoperative wound infections has prevented its widespread acceptance.

Nerve blocks

Injection of local anaesthetic near the nerve or nerves supplying the painful area may be useful after traumatic injury and for postoperative pain. Some examples of those commonly used include ring block for digital nerves, intercostal nerve blocks for pain relief after abdominal and thoracic surgical procedures, and femoral nerve block for pain after a fractured femur. (These are discussed in Chapter 13.) Similarly, individual nerves at the wrist or ankle may be blocked to provide areas of analgesia.

The peripheral nerves to the upper limb are invested in a connective tissue sheath and this anatomical arrangement has allowed the development of techniques that provide analgesia to the arm using blockade of the brachial plexus. Axillary*, supra-clavicular*, and interscalene* approaches to the brachial plexus sheath have been described and used for anaesthesia for surgical procedures and for postoperative analgesia. Prolonged analgesia can be maintained if a small catheter is placed into the sheath and used to administer repeated doses of local anaesthetic agents to maintain the blockade. A useful adjunct to this block is the local sympathetic blockade also produced, which may be beneficial in improving peripheral blood flow to the damaged limb or after surgical procedures involving the vasculature of the upper limb.

Field block

This technique involves the injection of local anaesthetic agent so as to create a zone of analgesia around the site of the wound. It may involve both nerve block and skin infiltration elements. This technique can be used to provide surgical anaesthesia for inguinal hernia repairs and also postoperative analgesia after such procedures.

Table 12.5 Choice of local anaesthetic agent

Procedure	Agent
Topical	
Bronchoscopy	Lignocaine 4%
ENT procedures	
Nasal operations	Cocaine
Oral	Benzocaine
Venepuncture	EMLA
Infiltration	
Wound	Lignocaine 0.5–1%
Fracture site	Bupivacaine 0.25%
	Prilocaine 0.5%
Nerve block	Lignocaine 1–2%
	Bupivacaine 0.25–0.5%
	Prilocaine 0.5–1%
Epidural	Lignocaine 1.5–2% with adrenaline (epinephrine)
	Bupivacaine 0.25–0.5%
	(Ropivacaine 0.5–1%)
Spinal	Bupivacaine 0.5% isobaric/hyperbaric

Epidural* and spinal* local analgesic blocks

Please refer to Chapters 14 to 16 inclusive.

Choice of local anaesthetic agent

Suitable local anaesthetic agents for the various techniques described are listed in Table 12.5

How to calculate the safe amount of local anaesthetic drug

The concentration of drug is usually derived from the weight of the drug and the volume of diluent (w/v). Thus, a 0.5% solution contains 0.5 g in 100 ml, or, 5 mg in 1 ml.

Example: A 70 kg patient needs to have a large laceration sutured on his scalp. How much of the various local anaesthetics can the doctor/nurse use?

For a 70 kg patient, the maximum safe doses of the various local anaesthetics are as listed in Table 12.3:

Bupivacaine	2 mg/kg	max safe dose = $2 \times 70 = 140$ mg
Lignocaine	3 mg/kg	max safe dose = $3 \times 70 = 210$ mg
Prilocaine	5 mg/kg	max safe dose = $5 \times 70 = 350$ mg

Assuming there is only 1% lignocaine available, the volume that can be used is:

1% lignocaine contains a concentration of 1 g in 100 ml. Which is the same as 1000 mg lignocaine in 100 ml = 10 mg lignocaine per ml. Therefore, the volume that can be safely used is 210 mg (the maximum safe dose calculated earlier) divided by the concentration available, i.e. 210/10 = 21 ml.

With adrenaline in 1 : 200 000 the maximum safe dose of lignocaine is 7 mg/kg, so the volume that can be used is:

Maximum safe dose for 70 kg person = $7 \times 70 = 490$ mg.
If 1% lignocaine (10 mg/ml) is available the volume that will contain this dose is 490/10 = 49 ml.

What if only 0.25% bupivacaine is available? The maximum safe dose for bupivacaine is 2 mg/kg, so for this 70 kg patient the dose would be 140 mg. 0.25% bupivacaine contains 0.25 g bupivacaine in one hundred ml. This is 250 mg in 100 ml = 2.5 mg per ml. Therefore, the volume of this concentration needed to achieve the maximum safe dose is 140/2.5 = 56 ml.

13

Local anaesthetic techniques

Some useful nerve blocks are described in this chapter. Not all of the techniques are suitable for readers of this book to perform but they are described to encourage understanding amongst those who may not be familiar with the methods, but who may have to care for patients before or after nerve blocks. Other blocks described may well be suitable for house officers to perform. This book complements more specialized instruction manuals and is not a substitute for adequate instruction in the practical points.

It is expected that before performing these nerve blocks, doctors will be proficient in resuscitation skills and that immediate access to resuscitation equipment, drugs, and assistance is available.

GENERAL CONTRAINDICATIONS TO LOCAL ANAESTHETIC PROCEDURES

1. Patient acceptance of any local anaesthetic technique is a prime consideration. Unwillingness to have any block performed should be accepted by the doctor, and the patient should not be pressurized into agreeing to the procedure. Anxiety about the procedure and risks can usually be allayed with adequate information and sensitive reassurance.
2. Sepsis at the proposed site of injection is a contraindication to all forms of local anaesthetic block. Spread of infection directly from the needle or intravascularly may result in abscess formation and morbidity. This is particularly important with techniques such as epidural or spinal blocks where the effects of abscesses may permanently damage spinal cord function.

3. Central nervous system or spinal disorders are often considered to be contraindications to epidural and spinal blocks. However, it is unlikely that these blocks affect the course of a chronic neurological disease such as multiple sclerosis.
4. Patients receiving anticoagulant therapy (warfarin or heparin) will be at greater risk of haematoma formation whatever block is used and advice over the suitability of the technique should be sought. Epidural and spinal blocks are contra-indicated.
5. Obesity and skeletal abnormalities may increase the difficulties associated with the performance of the block. Surface landmarks for deeper structures may be unreliable. Positioning the patient may also be difficult.

If difficulties are experienced in performing local analgesic techniques, do not persist, get help.

GENERAL PRINCIPLES OF REGIONAL ANAESTHESIA

1. Ask the patient about any previous exposure to local anaesthetic techniques and whether there were any complications of the procedure. Most often these are associated with dental procedures.
2. Examine the patient before performing a local anaesthetic block to ensure that you can identify the landmarks and there are no signs of sepsis at the proposed site of injection.
3. Explain the procedure to the patient, the expected effects, and the duration of the block. This is particularly important if temporary motor paralysis may occur with the nerve block or if prolonged sensory blockade may be experienced by the patient.
4. Note any concomitant medication that may influence your choice of technique.
5. All drugs and equipment required for performing the block should be assembled and checked.
6. Check that resuscitation equipment and drugs are available.

7. Before any block where potentially toxic doses of local anaesthetic agents may be administered or physiological effects such as hypotension resulting from the block itself may be expected, intravenous access should be obtained and secured. This enables rapid treatment of any adverse effects from the block or from systemic toxicity of the local anaesthetic agent used.

8. Before injecting any local anaesthetic always aspirate the syringe first. If blood is obtained do not inject the local anaesthetic. Even small amounts given intravenously can produce serious toxicity.

9. The patient should be monitored during the procedure. When epidural and spinal blocks are being performed this may include an ECG and automatic blood-pressure recordings to detect hypotension occurring as a result of the sympathetic blockade produced by the technique.

10. The patient should be positioned appropriately for the particular technique to be performed.

11. An aseptic technique must be used for all blocks. The person performing the nerve block should be scrubbed and wear sterile gloves. Gowns may be worn, in addition, when performing epidural and spinal blocks. The skin area where the nerve block will be performed should be cleaned with antiseptic solutions of iodine, chlorhexidine, or alcohol and covered with sterile drapes.

12. Communication should be maintained with the patient throughout the procedure. If parasthesiae are to be elicited to identify the position of the needle the patient should be warned to expect 'pins and needles' and their distribution. This should prevent inadvertent movement in response to these sensations which will reduce the risk of needle displacement. If any untoward effects such as tinnitus, dizziness, or pain with injection of the local anaesthetic are felt the patient should be asked to report them.

13. The early signs of systemic toxicity (see page 114) should be sought during injection of the local anaesthetic solution. If they occur stop the injection and begin appropriate treatment.

14. Observe the patient. Remember that no analgesic technique is 100 per cent effective all the time. Further analgesia or modification to the technique may be required.

WOUND INFILTRATION/INSTILLATION

Indications

- Postoperative analgesia: herniotomy, orchidopexy in children, herniorrhaphy in adults.
- Before suture: skin lacerations, episiotomy repairs.

Technique

Wound instillation is commonly carried out at the end of the operative procedure and may be performed at the closure of the wound at both deep and superficial levels. A suitable agent would be bupivacaine 0.25 per cent at doses of 0.5 ml/kg in children. Infiltration of local anaesthetic subcutaneously along the wound edges may be performed for anaesthesia before suturing of simple wounds or lacerations. It will provide analgesia after surgery.

DIGITAL NERVE BLOCK

Indications

Trauma: Before suturing of lacerations to fingers/toes.

- Surgery: local anaesthesia for surgical operations to fingers/toes.

Anatomy

The major digital nerves run on the ventrolateral aspects of the fingers/toes and are accompanied by the digital vessels. They give off articular branches and also a dorsal branch to supply the nail bed. In the hand these main nerves originate from the median and ulnar nerves; further small dorsal digital nerves originating from the radial nerve supply the dorsum of the fingers.

Technique

The digital nerves may be blocked at each side of the digit at the proximal phalanx. Injections of 1–2 ml of 2 per cent lignocaine should be made from the dorsal aspect, on each side, into the finger through skin weals using a 23 or 25 G needle. A further 1–2 ml may be infiltrated along the dorsal aspect of the digit between the two injection sites to ensure blockade of the dorsal branches. Analgesia may take 10–15 minutes to develop. This technique is suitable for minor surgical procedures such as toenail removal and suturing of lacerations.

INTERCOSTAL NERVE BLOCK

Indications

Trauma: rib fractures.

● Surgery: thoracic or abdominal.

Anatomy

The intercostal nerves run segmentally under the lower border of the respective ribs, between the external and internal intercostal muscles. They supply the intercostal muscles, transversus thoracis, and the abdominal muscles. They are sensory for the chest wall and abdomen. For analgesia of the abdominal wall, blockade of T5–T12 is required.

Technique

Intercostal nerve block is best performed in the mid-axillary line with the patient supine. The arm should be fully abducted and held anteriorly, elevating the scapula and allowing access to the inter-costal nerves from the fourth nerve downwards. The caudad margin of the rib should be palpated between the finger and thumb of the left hand and the overlying skin fixed. A 21 or 23 G needle attached to the syringe containing the local anaesthetic solution is inserted towards the rib aiming to make contact with the rib just above the caudad edge. Once this contact has been made the needle should be angulated in a caudad direction and gradually 'walked off the rib' to pass just under the caudad border of the rib. The needle should be advanced approximately 2–3 mm from the surface of the rib. Careful aspiration of the syringe at this time is essential. If blood is obtained (indicating intravascular placement of the needle) or air (indicating pleural penetration) the needle should be withdrawn. Should no air or blood be obtained at aspiration then 2.5 ml of bupivacaine 0.25 per cent should be injected at each intercostal space to be blocked. As the needle is withdrawn, a further 0.5 ml of local anaesthetic can be injected to anaesthetize the site of entry. This will ensure that when blocks need to be repeated less discomfort will be experienced.

Bupivacaine is the local anaesthetic of choice providing prolonged analgesia — up to 12 hours.

For midline abdominal wounds, complete analgesia following intercostal nerve blockade will require bilateral blocks.

Analgesia in the region of the xiphisternum will require blockade of the sixth to eighth intercostal nerves. To reach the umbilicus, blockade will need to extend to the tenth intercostal nerve (Fig. 13.1).

Alternatively the intercostal nerves may be blocked posteriorly at the angle of the ribs. This is performed with the patient in a lateral position and the injection points are lateral to the erector spinae muscles, approximately 8 cm from the midline. Again the procedure should be to advance the needle until it slips under the caudad border of the rib, where 2–3 ml of bupivacaine should be injected after careful aspiration for blood and air. The patient's arms may need to be elevated across the chest to allow access to the sixth and seventh intercostal nerves by elevating the scapula. Bilateral blocks will require the patient to be turned to allow access to the opposite side.

Complications

The most important complication is the development of a pneumothorax resulting from lung puncture. Usually this is minor and will resolve spontaneously. Occasionally a tension pneumothorax may be produced and will require immediate insertion of an underwater-seal chest drain. If air is aspirated at any time during the performance of the blocks, an erect chest X-ray should be performed to detect the presence of a pneumothorax. Bilateral intereostal nerve blockade risks bilateral pneumothoraces and must only be undertaken by experienced clinicians aware of the risk.

Care should be taken not to exceed the maximum doses of local

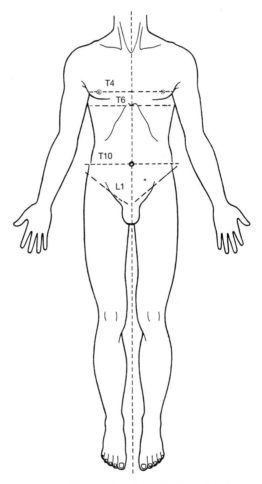

Fig. 13.1 Landmarks for levels of analgesia after intercostal nerve blockade.

anaesthetic when multiple blocks are to be performed. Local anaesthetic is absorbed rapidly following intercostal nerve block because of the high vascularity of this region. Preparations containing adrenaline (epinephrine) may be used to reduce absorption, and careful aspiration should be performed with each injection to prevent intravascular administration and systemic local anaesthetic toxicity.

FEMORAL NERVE BLOCK

Indications

- Fractured shaft of femur.
- Surgery/trauma to thigh and knee.
- Surgery/trauma to lower leg (in combination with sciatic nerve blockade).

Femoral nerve block is ideally suited for the immediate care of patients with fractures of the shaft of the femur. Good analgesia is produced within 10 minutes and enables the patient to be examined and X-rayed with minimal discomfort. Good motor blockade from bupivacaine also reduces painful muscle spasm that is commonly associated with the fracture.

Anatomy

The femoral nerve runs from the lumbar plexus between the psoas and iliac muscles and enters the thigh by passing deep to the inguinal ligament. It innervates the skin of the anterior thigh and medial side of the calf down to the medial malleolus. It also has branches to the quadriceps muscles and sartorius muscle, and supplies the knee joint.

Technique

The femoral nerve is accessible, just below the inguinal ligament, lateral to the femoral arterial pulse.

Standing on the opposite side to that on which the block is to be performed, the pulsation of the femoral artery should be palpated just below the inguinal ligament. The injection site is 1–2 cm lateral to the femoral artery and the needle should be directed cephalad. Parasthesia may be obtained in the conscious patient indicating the correct position of the needle. In unconscious patients the injection should be made in a fan-like manner to a depth of 3–5 cm, aspirating at each injection. If firm digital pressure is maintained distal to the injection site, local anaesthetic in the neurovascular sheath will be directed cephalad, blocking the obturator nerve and the lateral femoral cutaneous nerve of the thigh. This is the so-called '3-in-1' block.

Bupivacaine 0.25 or 0.5 per cent are the local anaesthetic agents of choice for this block. In adults, volumes of 20 ml should be used. When the 3-in-1 block is performed, 30 ml of local anaesthetic solution may be required.

14

An introduction to epidural and spinal analgesia

Epidurals and spinals are techniques of blocking pain transmission at nerve root and spinal cord level. Though both techniques offer good pain relief, there are a number of important differences between the techniques which need to be appreciated as these affect how the patient is managed. The differences are listed in Table 14.1.

Epidurals involve the placement of a catheter through a needle inserted in the epidural space just outside the dura mater. Through this catheter, continuous infusions of analgesic agents can be given. In spinals, a fine needle is inserted from the skin through the dura and arachnoid mater into the subarachnoid space to enable injection of the analgesic agents directly into the cerebrospinal fluid. Relative to epidurals, small volumes of analgesic agents are needed

Table 14.1 Differences between epidurals and spinals

Epidural	Spinal
Time-consuming to perform (10–20 min)	Quick to perform (2–5 min)
Onset of analgesia takes 10–20 min	Quick onset of analgesia (2–3 min)
Risk of local anaesthetic toxicity because of large amounts needed	Minimal risk of local anaesthetic toxicity as small amounts used
Risk of patchy block	Consistent block, rarely patchy analgesia
Can be used for continuous analgesia via a catheter	Usually a single-shot technique; continuous catheter techniques of analgesia are controversial
Typical dose: 10–15 ml of 0.5% bupivacaine	Typical dose: 2–3 ml of 0.5% bupivacaine

for spinal analgesia as they do not have to penetrate the dura and arachnoid mater. In addition, little is lost to systemic absorption or leakage from the site of injection. Figure 14.1 illustrates the different end points of the epidural catheter and spinal needle.

Though the mainstay of epidural and spinal analgesia involves the use of local anaesthetics and opioids, midazolam, clonidine, and ketamine have also been used for their analgesic effects.

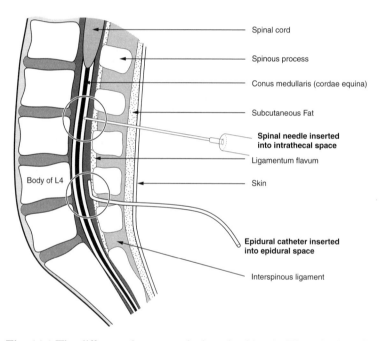

Fig. 14.1 The difference between spinals and epidurals. The spinal needle is inserted into the intrathecal space which contains CSF bathing the cordae equinae and spinal cord. Very small amounts of local anaesthetic injected here will spread widely and easily bind to nerve tissue to block conduction. The epidural catheter is inserted through a large needle into the epidural space which lies outside the dural layer which surrounds the CSF and spinal cord. The epidural space usually contains fat and a few blood vessels and because it is more distant from nerve tissue, larger amounts of local anaesthetic are needed to produce analgesia equivalent to that of the spinal.

There are a number of similarities between epidurals and spinals:

- Mechanism of analgesia: both involve reversible blockade of nerve conduction at spinal cord and nerve root level.
- Sequence of nerve block: the effects of local anaesthetic agents on nerve conduction are seen first on the smaller diameter fibres — pre-ganglionic sympathetic fibres being the most easily blocked. Sensory modalities are blocked in the order of increasing fibre diameter — temperature, pain, touch, and pressure. The final level of blockade is of the motor and proprioception pathways.
- Technique: both involve insertion of a needle in the back but to different end points. Spinal needles tend to be very fine (22–27G) and are intentionally inserted until free cerebrospinal fluid (CSF) drainage occurs, whereas the epidural needle (usually much larger, 16–18G) is inserted into the epidural space, carefully avoiding any CSF leak.
- Complications: a postdural puncture headache can occur after either procedure as can an epidural or spinal haematoma resulting in paraperesis. Infection can be introduced resulting in an epidural abscess or meningitis. Occasionally trauma to nerve roots can occur during needle insertion resulting in pins and needles or localized increased sensitivity to pain that can persist for days or weeks.
- Contraindications to either procedure include:
  - bleeding tendency;
  - local sepsis at site of epidural;
  - hypotension;
  - raised intracranial pressure;
  - acute neurological conditions;
  - patient refusal.
- Relative contraindications:
  - difficult anatomy.

When properly performed, in a well-selected patient, the techniques enable patients to undergo operations without sedation (for example, transurethral resection of prostate), to recover from major surgery without pain (for example, abdominal aortic aneurysm repair), and to regain the ability to cough and clear secretions in spite of abdominal incisions (particularly important in patients with chest infections.)

Whatever the indication when epidurals or spinals are used for analgesia, the level of analgesia sensory blockade must cover the extent of the incision at least, and ideally be two segments higher to ensure good pain relief. The different levels of neural blockade required for different operations are outlined in Table 14.2.

Table 14.2 Levels of spinal and epidural anaesthesia required for surgical procedures

Level of blockade	Type of surgery
T4–5 (nipple)	Upper abdominal e.g. gastrectomy
T6–8 (xiphisternum)	Intestinal, gynaecological, and urological
T10 (umbilicus)	Transurethral resection of prostrate, obstetric vaginal delivery, Hip
L1 (inguinal ligament)	Thigh, lower limb amputations
L2–3 (knee and below)	Foot
S2–5 (perineal)	Haemorrhoidectomy, other perineal

OPIOIDS VERSUS LOCAL ANAESTHETICS

With local anaesthetics, the epidural catheter must be sited close to the area in which the blockade is required. The local anaesthetic may be given either by continuous infusion (with a risk of increasing levels of block) or by repeated top-up doses (with risks of episodes of hypotension or acute toxicity). Experienced staff are required to carry out repeat injections and to deal with the adverse effects.

Opioid drugs will provide a longer duration of analgesia, without the attendant risks of hypotension, and have a greater spread. Catheters sited in the lumbar region can still give analgesia in the upper abdomen and chest and as they are technically easier to insert than those in the thoracic region, there is therefore reduced risk of spinal cord injury. There is no motor blockade and other sensory modalities are unaffected with the opioids. However, all opioid drugs have potential for producing delayed (4–24 hours) respiratory depression. The main differences between opioids and local anaesthetics when used in spinals and epidurals are listed in Table 14.3.

Table 14.3 Effects of epidural/intrathecal opioids vs. local anaesthetics

Opioid	Local anaesthetic
Partial blockade of pain perception (no motor or other sensory blockade)	Full blockade of all sensory and motor nerve impulses
No autonomic blockade	Autonomic blockade, so hypotension common
Needs to be used with local anaesthetics for complete anaesthesia	Can be used alone for complete anaesthesia
Side-effects: nausea and vomiting (by stimulating vomiting centre); itching (not histamine mediated); respiratory depression	Side-effects: shivering

NOVEL SPINAL ANALGESIC AGENTS

Clonidine

This is an adrenergic receptor agonist drug which is primarily used in the treatment of hypertension. However, when given into the epidural or subarachnoid space in experimental animals, this drug also produces analgesia. The analgesic effects are believed to result from pre- and postsynaptic receptor activation in the spinal cord which may block pain transmission by inhibiting the release of the neurotransmitter substance P and by reducing the activity of dorsal horn neurones.

Ketamine

This is an anaesthetic induction agent that has analgesic properties when given intravenously or into the epidural and subarachnoid space. It is believed to act by blocking the NMDA (N-methyl D-aspartate) receptor which is an excitatory ion channel coupled receptor implicated in anaesthesia and analgesia.

COMMON COMPLICATIONS

Hypotension

This may occur as a result of the blockade of the sympathetic fibres producing vasodilatation in the area of the block. This should be treated with ephedrine (3–5 mg boluses IV) and intravenous volume expansion (1–21 of 0.9 per cent saline).

Hypotension is accentuated in the pregnant patient particularly when lying supine. This results from the aorto-caval compression from the gravid uterus. Hypotensive pregnant patients should therefore always be turned on to their sides and intravenous fluids and vasopressors administered if this manoeuvre does not improve the blood pressure.

Postdural puncture headache

Headache can be one of the most disabling complications after spinal blocks (where the dura is breached deliberately) or after epidural blocks (where the dura is breached accidentally). The incidence of accidental dural punctures during epidural insertion is 1%. The frequency of the headache is related to the size and design of the needle tip penetrating the dura. Larger needles with cutting tips have a greater incidence of headache than smaller needles with blunt tips (see Table 14.4).

The headache usually occurs within one to four days of the procedure and is made worse by the upright position and by coughing and straining. The pain is usually located in the occipital region and may be associated with neck stiffness. It is believed to be related to the leak of cerebrospinal fluid through the dura and efforts to reduce the incidence of headache have centred around

Table 14.4 Relationship between incidence of postdural puncture headache and needle size (Nb: 16G needle is *larger* than 26G needle)

Needle size (G)	Tip type	Incidence of headache (%)
16	Cutting	75
20	Cutting	30
25	Blunt	1.1
26	Cutting	5–7

the use of smaller needles to reduce the dural puncture size. The headache may last for one to two weeks but there are occasional reports of it persisting for months.

Management of postdural puncture headache

1. Give adequate, regular simple analgesics, such as paracetamol or other NSAIDs.
2. Maintain hydration — regular oral fluids or, if the patient is unable to take oral fluids, then the intravenous route should be used.
3. Avoidance of coughing and straining — stool-softening agents or laxatives such as lactulose may be useful.
4. Bed rest is usually necessary simply because the headache is worse when the patient is upright.
5. The anaesthetist responsible for performing the block should be informed. He or she will then be able to reassure the patient and monitor the response to the simple measures just described. If, despite these measures, the headache persists, the anaesthetist may then inject 10–20 ml of the patient's own blood into the epidural space to stop the CSF leak ('epidural blood patch'). This technique is usually rapidly effective in 70 to 80 per cent of cases.

Alternative therapies to alleviate the headache include the use of large doses of caffeine, either orally or intravenously. Although this has been successful in some cases it may provide only temporary improvement.

EXTREMELY RARE COMPLICATIONS

Spinal/epidural haematoma

The risk of spinal and epidural haematomas is extremely low — estimates are 1:150 000 from epidural procedures and 1:220 000 from spinal procedures in patients with normal coagulation. The main symptoms are severe back pain and loss of sphincter control. It needs surgical management (decompression laminectomy) within eight hours of onset for chance of full recovery. The risk will be higher in patients on aspirin, minidose standard heparin, or minidose low molecular weight heparin. Suggested guidelines about coagulopathies are given in Table 14.5.

Table 14.5 Summary of recommendations for neuraxial procedures when a patient may have coagulopathy

Haemostatic status	Safety measures
Minor haemostatic abnormality	
Aspirin	Discontinue for >5 days if heparin anticoagulation anticipated (e.g. cardiac/vascular surgery)
Minidose standard heparin	Perform procedures *including removal of catheter* at least 1 h before next dose or 4–6 h after most recent dose
Minidose LMW heparin	Perform procedure *including removal of catheter* at least 2 h before next dose or 12 h after most recent dose
Thrombocytopaenia	Individualize risks and potential benefits for platelets if count $50–100 \times 10^9/L$; no concerns with higher counts
Major haemostatic abnormality	
Intraoperative heparin therapy	Delay heparin therapy at least 1 h after block; *do not remove epidural catheter until heparin effect resolved*; consider aborting anticoagulation if bloody tap occurred
Full anticoagulation (heparin/ warfarin)	Procedures are contraindicated; reverse anticoagulation
Thrombolytic therapy	No data; procedures contraindicated

(Reproduced with permission from *Can J Anaes* (1996) **43:**5 R129- 35)

Epidural abscess/meningitis

These are even rarer and usually arise due to breakdown of aseptic technique and occasionally from bacteraemia unrelated to epidural insertion technique. The presenting features tend to be similar to that of a haematoma but generally include a fever and signs of meningism. Once the diagnosis is confirmed by an MRI/CT scan, the treatment ordinarily involves surgical drainage and antibiotics.

15

Spinal anaesthesia

The earliest reported use of spinal anaesthesia in man was by August Bier, in 1898, who injected cocaine intrathecally. The technique was further developed and used widely with newer local anaesthetic agents. Fears of neurological complications following spinal anaesthesia led to a decline in its popularity in the UK in the 1950s. These fears have since been felt to be unjustified. Spinal anaesthesia is now recognized as a safe and effective technique. It is principally used to provide anaesthesia for surgical procedures below the umbilicus, particularly for orthopaedic and urological operations.

With most of the currently available local anaesthetic agents for spinal use, the blockade produced is of relatively short duration and provides little postoperative analgesia. Techniques using the insertion of catheters into the subarachnoid space can offer analgesia by continuous administration of local anaesthetic providing a prolonged block. Since the catheters must be inserted intrathecally and may give a portal of entry for bacteria this technique is not, so far, widely used.

The extent of blockade achieved after subarachnoid injection of local anaesthetic agents depends on a number of factors.

1. *Specific gravity of local anaesthetic solutions.* Local anaesthetic agents for spinal use have been prepared in solutions of differing specific gravity with respect to CSF. Solutions are available as isobaric, hypobaric, and hyperbaric forms when they are the same, less, or more dense than CSF respectively. Hyperbaric solutions will tend to produce more profound effects in the more dependent regions, in contrast to hypobaric solutions where the effects will be more concentrated in the uppermost regions.

2. *Patient position* during and after injection of the local anaesthetic solution. Sitting a patient up may produce a more profound block in the sacral roots when a hyperbaric solution is used.
3. *Site of injection.* Blockade will be produced more rapidly and more extensively in regions close to the site of injection. In addition, the curvatures of the spine in the thoracic and lumbar regions will tend to limit the spread of solution injected at distal sites and therefore limit the extent of the block.
4. *Volume and dose of drug injected.* The extent of blockade will be greater with both larger doses of drug and greater volumes injected into the CSF.

Suitable agents are listed in Table 15.1. By combining the particular preparation with posture it is possible to influence the spread of local anaesthetic blockade. Examples include the following:

Saddle block

Typically this utilizes a hyperbaric local anaesthetic solution injected in a low lumbar interspace with the patient in a sitting position. This leads to the development of a block principally in the sacral region, making it suitable for operations in the region of distribution of the sacral nerve roots such as haemorrhoidectomy.

Unilateral block

This technique again uses hyperbaric anaesthetic solution. A predominantly unilateral block is obtained by injection with the patient lying on the side that is to be anaesthetized. Alternatively, if a hypobaric solution is used the principal effects of the block would be on the uppermost side.

Table 15.1 Local anaesthetic agents for spinal blocks

Agent	Dose for block to T10	Dose for block to T4	Duration of block (min)
Bupivacaine 0.5% isobaric	10–15 mg (2–3 ml)	15–20 mg (3–4 ml)	150–200
Bupivacaine 0.5% hyperbaric	15 mg (3 ml)	20 mg (4 ml)	90 –110

16

Epidural analgesia

Epidural analgesia is an invasive procedure which has a number of benefits. It provides optimal analgesia for operations on the lower limbs, abdomen, and thorax and allows effective chest physiotherapy in the presence of abdominal and chest incisions. It also minimizes the sympathetic stimulation of the heart which in turn decreases the oxygen demand of the heart and may decrease myocardial ischaemia. By avoiding the need for intravenous and intramuscular opioids, the epidural minimizes the sedative and respiratory depressant effects of these drugs and allows earlier return of gut function. In obstetrics, it provides optimal analgesia for labour which can be easily supplemented for a caesarian section, thus avoiding the risks of emergency general anaesthesia.

Indications for:

Lumbar epidurals: lower abdominal/lower limb surgery; obstetric analgesia/anaesthesia.

Thoracic epidurals: upper abdominal surgery/thoracic surgery; chest trauma.

ANATOMY OF THE EPIDURAL SPACE

The epidural space is a loose connective tissue-filled area between the outer layer of the spinal dura and the vertebral canal. It extends from the foramen magnum to the sacral hiatus. The contents of the space include the dural sac and spinal nerve roots, the epidural venous plexus, and the spinal arteries, lymphatic vessels, and fat.

The average width of the space is 0.5 cm. It is at its largest in the lumbar region.

SITE OF ACTION OF INJECTED AGENTS

When a solution of local anaesthetic agent is injected into the epidural space its effects are exerted either on nerve roots in the epidural or paravertebral spaces or intradurally after diffusion through the dura into the subarachnoid space. An analgesic solution injected into the epidural space may spread caudally and cephalad, extending the region of blockade.

TECHNIQUE

The principle involves the detection of the sudden loss of resistance as the epidural needle is advanced into the epidural space. The loss of resistance is best detected at the plunger of a syringe (filled with air or 0.9 per cent saline) attached to the end of the epidural needle which is kept under pressure by the anaesthetist's hand while at the same time advancing the epidural needle. On entering the epidural space saline or air can be injected because the needle is being advanced by pressure on the plunger of the syringe, the sudden ease of injection stops the movement of the needle. If the needle is advanced a millimetre too far (after entering the epidural space), a dural puncture may occur followed by a severe headache.

After insertion of the epidural needle into the epidural space, a catheter is threaded through the needle and the needle removed leaving the catheter in place. Before starting the epidural infusion the catheter is aspirated to detect CSF or blood which would indicate intrathecal or intravascular placement of the catheter respectively. If either of these occur, the local analgesic should not be given and the epidural should be aborted or re-inserted.

Once the local analgesic has been given, the development of the block can be monitored by both sensory loss (using ice or a pinprick) and motor weakness (inability to raise the legs).

PATIENT MONITORING

Intravenous access must be maintained in all patients until the effects of the block have worn off. Regular monitoring of the patient is important to ensure adequate levels of analgesia and, when using infusion techniques, that these levels do not extend progressively higher. High blocks may result in severe hypotension or breathing difficulties if the phrenic nerve (supplies the diaphragm) is blocked at its origins in the neck. Repeated checks of blood pressure are mandatory and must be performed at frequent intervals after each top-up bolus dose to detect any hypotension developing from sympathetic blockade.

Guidelines used at Addenbrooke's Hospital, Cambridge, for ward staff looking after a patient with an epidural infusion are given in Fig. 16.1; the nursing observations are recorded on the chart shown in Fig. 16.2.

MANAGEMENT OF AN EPIDURAL BLOCK

Factors that may influence the extent of spread of the local anaesthetic agent in the epidural space include the following:

1. *Volume of local anaesthetic solution:* although the total dose of drug administered is of major importance, the concentration — and thereby the volume — in which this is administered may also influence the extent of the block, although this is often unpredictable. In general the extent of the block may be greater if the same mass of drug is injected in a greater volume of solution.
2. *Patient age*: the elderly require less drug than the young to produce the same extent of blockade.
3. *Pregnancy*: less local anaesthetic is required to produce a similar extent of blockade in pregnant patients compared with the non-pregnant state.
4. *Site of injection*: spread of local anaesthetic produces a more extensive blockade after injection in the thoracic region compared with the lumbar region.
5. *Local anaesthetic agent used*: different local anaesthetic agents can produce blockades of different extent and nature. Etidocaine produces a more profound motor block than bupivacaine.

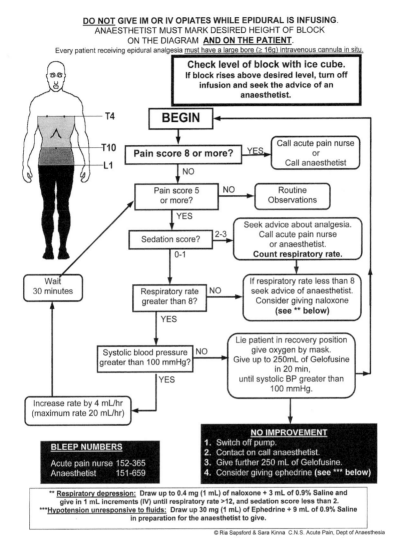

DO NOT GIVE IM OR IV OPIATES WHILE EPIDURAL IS INFUSING.
ANAESTHETIST MUST MARK DESIRED HEIGHT OF BLOCK
ON THE DIAGRAM **AND ON THE PATIENT**.
Every patient receiving epidural analgesia must have a large bore (≥ 16g) intravenous cannula in situ.

Check level of block with ice cube.
If block rises above desired level, turn off infusion and seek the advice of an anaesthetist.

T4
T10
L1

BEGIN

Pain score 8 or more? — YES → Call acute pain nurse or Call anaesthetist

NO

Pain score 5 or more? — NO → Routine Observations

YES

Sedation score? — 2-3 → Seek advice about analgesia. Call acute pain nurse or anaesthetist. **Count respiratory rate.**

0-1

Wait 30 minutes

Respiratory rate greater than 8? — NO → If respiratory rate less than 8 seek advice of anaesthetist. Consider giving naloxone **(see ** below)**

YES

Systolic blood pressure greater than 100 mmHg? — NO → Lie patient in recovery position give oxygen by mask. Give up to 250mL of Gelofusine in 20 min, until systolic BP greater than 100 mmHg.

YES

Increase rate by 4 mL/hr (maximum rate 20 mL/hr)

BLEEP NUMBERS
Acute pain nurse 152-365
Anaesthetist   151-659

NO IMPROVEMENT
1. Switch off pump.
2. Contact on call anaesthetist.
3. Give further 250 mL of Gelofusine.
4. Consider giving ephedrine **(see *** below)**

** Respiratory depression: Draw up to 0.4 mg (1 mL) of naloxone + 3 mL of 0.9% Saline and give in 1 mL increments (IV) until respiratory rate >12, and sedation score less than 2.
***Hypotension unresponsive to fluids: Draw up 30 mg (1 mL) of Ephedrine + 9 mL of 0.9% Saline in preparation for the anaesthetist to give.

© Ria Sapsford & Sara Kinna C.N.S. Acute Pain, Dept of Anaesthesia

Fig. 16.1 Guidelines for epidural infusions. The infusion is prescribed by a preprinted sticker. (0.1% Bupivacaine with 2 μg/ml of Fentanyl.)

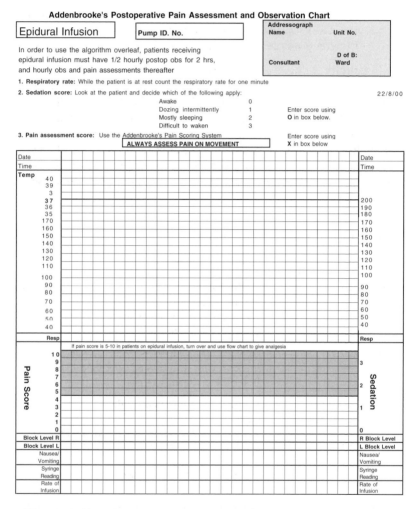

Addenbrooke's Postoperative Pain Assessment and Observation Chart

Epidural Infusion		Pump ID. No.		Addressograph Name	Unit No.

In order to use the algorithm overleaf, patients receiving
epidural infusion must have 1/2 hourly postop obs for 2 hrs,
and hourly obs and pain assessments thereafter

1. **Respiratory rate:** While the patient is at rest count the respiratory rate for one minute

2. **Sedation score:** Look at the patient and decide which of the following apply:

Awake	0	
Dozing intermittently	1	Enter score using
Mostly sleeping	2	**O** in box below.
Difficult to waken	3	

22/8/00

3. **Pain assessment score:** Use the <u>Addenbrooke's Pain Scoring System</u>
   ALWAYS ASSESS PAIN ON MOVEMENT

Enter score using
X in box below

Fig. 16.2 Chart for recording the nursing observations of patients with epidurals.

6. *Positioning of the patient*: position during and immediately after the injection affects the spread of blockade in a similar manner to spinal anaesthesia.

7. *Amount of local anaesthetic agent*: overall, effects of the block are related to the total dose of drug administered. In children,

doses may be calculated on a mg/kg basis and when the caudal route is used as access to the epidural space in children these doses can produce predictable blockade.

For prolonged analgesia a catheter is inserted into the epidural space allowing repeated administration of local anaesthetic. Bupivacaine is the most commonly used local anaesthetic for epidural blockade. Incremental doses of 5–10 ml of 0.25 or 0.5 per cent solutions may be given intermittently to maintain an appropriate level of analgesia. Alternatively a continuous infusion of local anaesthetic solution may be given. Some of the problems that may be encountered with epidural infusions and suggested solutions are outlined in Table 16.1

Table 16.1 Troubleshooting epidurals

Problem	Solutions to consider
No analgesia	Pump malfunctioning Syringe empty Loose connection allowing leakage Catheter displaced
Patchy block	Give top up and increase infusion rate Increase concentration of local anaesthetic Pull back catheter by 1 cm
Unilateral block/ missed segment	Lie patient on unblocked side Give top up Try top up after pulling back catheter by 1 cm

EPIDURAL CATHETERS

These are 20 gauge catheters that can be placed in the epidural space and through which intermittent injections or infusions of local anaesthetic agents can be given. They can have a single end hole or multiple holes with a rounded end. There is debate as to how long a catheter may be left in the epidural space. Ideally they should be removed after 72 hours (as this is the recommended effective life of the antimicrobial filters); after five days the incidence of complications with epidurals starts to increase dramatically. There have been reports of catheters being in place for up to two weeks without difficulties. It is important that strict adherence to asepsis occurs while siting the epidural.

Catheters should be removed with gentle traction at the skin entry site. Once removed the catheter must be checked to ensure that it has all been removed. If, during removal, resistance is felt, gentle continuous traction with the spine flexed may help. Generally only 2–4 cm of catheter are left in the epidural space and the risk of knots in the catheter is low. If continued difficulty is experienced, the catheter may have caught around a nerve root in which case the patient will complain of pain when traction is applied to the catheter. Should this occur the catheter should be left in position and radiographs taken with contrast injected through the catheter to localize its position. If it is located in the vicinity of a nerve root, removal by formal laminectomy may be necessary.

If on removal the catheter is found to have fractured, leaving small amounts in the epidural space, this should be recorded in the patient's notes and the patient informed. Small fragments are unlikely to require surgical removal and may prove difficult to locate if laminectomy is performed.

Catheter removal in patients with coagulopathies

Evidence is accumulating that catheter removal can be as dangerous as the procedure itself in patients who are on prophylactic heparin (both standard and low molecular weight) to protect against deep vein thrombosis and pulmonary embolis. Thus catheter removal must be carefully timed (see Table 14.5, page 136).

EPIDURAL TOP-UP PROCEDURES

These are suggested instructions that may be left for nurses when epidurals are managed by them. Epidurals using local anaesthetic agents should not be routinely managed on general wards but only in high-dependency or intensive care units because of the hazards involved.

1. Check prescription and volume and concentration of local anaesthetic.

2. Check the level of sensory block still present and if remaining high while the patient is in pain call the doctor/anaesthetist for advice.
3. Check that the intravenous infusion is running.
4. Aspirate the epidural catheter, looking for evidence of blood or free flow of CSF.
5. Give 3 ml of the local anaesthetic as a small test dose and monitor for high block or hypotension.
6. Give the remainder of the dose slowly if no complications have occurred after the initial dose.
7. Ensure appropriate monitoring of the patient — blood pressure, level of block — at 5- minute intervals for 30 minutes after each top-up.

COMMON COMPLICATIONS

(See Chapter 14)

- Postdural puncture headaches. (Occurs in ~1% of epidural insertions.)
- Hypotension may occur as a result of the blockade of the sympathetic fibres producing vasodilatation.

RARE COMPLICATIONS

- Intravascular administration of local anaesthetic will result in the signs and symptoms of systemic local anaesthetic toxicity (see Chapter 12).
- Accidental subarachnoid administration of local anaesthetic will result in the extension of the block to high levels, usually following a bolus (top-up) dose. It may occur through inadvertent, unrecognized dural puncture at the time of performing the block, or some time after if the catheter has migrated through the dura. The clinical features are:
  Cardiovascular: hypotension occurs secondary to peripheral vasodilatation induced by sympathetic blockade. Bradycardia may result from blockage of cardiac sympathetic fibres from T1–4.

Respiratory: breathing difficulties occur with blocks above T4 as intercostal muscles are affected. This may be worsened by blocks at C3–5 when diaphragmatic paralysis occurs.

CNS: initially there is extensive sensory and motor blockade. Tingling and numbness in the hands indicates a rising block. Coma can occur if sufficient local anaesthetic reaches the brain stem.

Management:

- Explain to patient what is happening
- Give oxygen
- Sedate, intubate the trachea, and ventilate the lungs if respiratory compromise severe
- Support circulation with colloids, ephedrine, and atropine
- Transfer to intensive care

No harm should come to the patient if this is managed properly.

CAUDAL APPROACH TO THE EPIDURAL SPACE

The epidural space may also be approached through the sacral hiatus. This is a particularly useful route for producing blockade of the lower sacral nerve roots. It is used for perineal surgery or for postoperative analgesia following procedures such as haemorrhoidectomy. It is widely used in children, when the sacral hiatus is easily accessible, and provides analgesia following circumcision, orchidopexy, and herniotomy.

17

Epidural and intrathecal opioids

INTRODUCTION

Experiments in animals have shown the effect of small doses of opioid drugs on nociceptive transmission at the spinal cord level. Transmission of impulses from noxious stimuli upwards to the brain was inhibited. When chronic spinal catheterization was performed in animals intrathecal administration of opioids produced significant and long-lasting increases in nociceptive thresholds using thermal, electrical, and mechanical pain stimuli.

Spinal effects of opioid drugs result from alterations in pain transmission at the level of the first- and second-order neurones in the dorsal grey matter. Receptors for the opioid drugs are located in the substantia gelatinosa in the vicinity of the primary afferent terminals. Activation of opioid receptors results in hyperpolarization of the cell preventing excitation and its ability to conduct pain invoking signals.

When used in humans, the benefits of epidural or intrathecal opioid analgesia compared with that produced by local anaesthetic agents (see Table 14.3, page 133) administered by the same routes include the achievement of analgesia without sensory or motor deficit and, as a result of the lack of autonomic blockade, analgesia without the risks of hypotension. In addition, analgesic synergism between local analgesics and opioids given epidurally or intrathecally will decrease the concomitant dose of opioid required by these routes and may decrease the incidence of respiratory depression when compared to intravenous and intramuscular opioids.

INDICATIONS AND USES OF EPIDURAL OPIOIDS

- *Postoperative pain*: epidurals can provide analgesia after thoracic, upper, and lower abdominal surgery and also after orthopaedic procedures on the lower limbs.
- *Obstetrics*: epidural opioids provide analgesia both after Caesarean section operations and also in labour. Small doses of fentanyl will reduce the requirements for epidural local analgesic agents during the first stage of labour.
- *Trauma*: analgesia for rib fractures and limb injuries can be provided successfully using epidural opioids.

FACTORS INFLUENCING THE ACTION OF INTRATHECAL AND EPIDURAL OPIOIDS

Lipid solubility

The degree of lipid solubility of the agent determines the rate of penetration through lipid membranes and this will influence the onset of analgesia. The most lipid-soluble drugs (for example, fentanyl) will have a quicker onset of analgesia as a result of more rapid penetration into the neural tissue. However, the duration of action will be reduced as these drugs will be most rapidly cleared after absorption into the blood vessels. The slow onset of analgesia with a less lipid-soluble drug, such as morphine, is thought to be related to slow penetration into the spinal cord and sequestration of drug in the CSF.

Elimination

The duration of effects of the drugs will be influenced by the rate at which they are cleared from their sites of action. The endogenous opioid peptides are rapidly metabolized by peptidase enzymes in the CSF; exogenous opioid drugs are normally eliminated after absorption into the blood.

Route of administration

Drugs administered by the epidural route must penetrate the dura in addition to passing through the neural tissue, resulting in a delayed onset of action. Drugs may be absorbed from the epidural site into the fat normally present in this region and from there eliminated via the epidural venous plexus. Higher plasma concentrations are achieved after epidural administration compared to the intrathecal route.

UNWANTED EFFECTS

The nature and incidence of unwanted effects after epidural and intrathecal administration of opioids remain the major factors limiting the use of these techniques. The most serious complication is respiratory depression, although the minor sequelae of pruritis, nausea and vomiting, and urinary retention are common and distressing.

Central nervous system effects

The typical central nervous system effects of opioids such as euphoria, sedation, and respiratory depression still occur when epidural and intrathecal routes are used. This has been taken as evidence that opioids, when administered intrathecally or epidurally, reach higher centres. This may be the result of drug redistribution by the blood following absorption from the CSF or as a result of bulk flow within the CSF.

Early central nervous system effects are thought to result from drug distribution after vascular uptake, whereas the late effects may result from CSF transfer. Late effects are most commonly seen with morphine which, because of its low lipid solubility, persists in the CSF in appreciable quantity.

Peripheral effects

Pruritus

Pruritus occurs after both epidural and intrathecal administration, although widely differing rates have been reported — some studies suggest that this complication occurs in up to two-thirds of the patients who receive morphine. Itching is also associated with fentanyl, diamorphine, and pethidine administration, although the incidence is lower than with morphine. Itching is unrelated to histamine release or to the dose of drug used. It is usually unrelated to the segmental area of action of the opioid drug and occurs frequently around the head and neck. It may be severe and prolonged and may last up to 30 hours after morphine administration.

Pruritus may be relieved by the systemic administration of small doses of naloxone (0.1 mg). This does not adversely affect analgesia.

Nausea and vomiting

Nausea and vomiting are associated with the use of opioids, whatever route is employed. The incidence after epidural and intrathecal administration is between 30 and 50 per cent.

Urinary retention

Urinary retention is variable with an incidence of 30–40 per cent. It occurs more commonly in males and is increased after intrathecal compared with epidural administration. The mechanism by which this occurs is unclear. Since minimal effects on bladder function are seen after systemic opioid use, this adverse effect must be caused by the high concentrations produced around the spinal cord, affecting bladder-control mechanisms. The effects may be prolonged (up to 14–16 hours) although they may be relieved by systemic administration of naloxone.

Respiratory depression

Respiratory depression is a major concern when intrathecal and epidural opioids are used, particularly since it may occur some time (up to 24 hours) after the drug has been given (see Table 17.1).

Table 17.1 Incidence of respiratory depression after epidural opioids

Drug	Dose	Time occurring
Morphine	2–10 mg	4–22 h
Diamorphine	2–10 mg	20 min – 4.5 h
Pethidine	50–100 mg	5–30 min
Methadone	4–6 mg	20 min – 4 h
Fentanyl	0.1 µg	30 min – 4 h

Adapted from Morgan (1989)

There appear to be several groups of patients who are at increased risk, including the elderly and those who have received systemic opioids or other central nervous system depressant drugs (such as benzodiazepines).

The less lipid-soluble opioids are most likely to cause this complication as a large reservoir of drug remains in the CSF and may be distributed to higher centres. Administration of opioid into the epidural space in the thoracic region or intrathecal administration also appears to increase the risk. Large doses by either route will further increase the risks of this complication.

Naloxone will reverse the respiratory depression but repeated doses or infusions may be needed for the prolonged period during which the patient remains at risk after intrathecal and epidural administration.

THE IDEAL AGENT FOR SPINALS AND EPIDURALS

Opinions vary on this. Some authors feel such agents should have:

- high lipid solubility, which will produce rapid passage of the drug through the dura, permitting epidural use. High lipid solubility will enable rapid absorption of the drug from the spinal depot and reduce the risks of delayed respiratory depression;
- high affinity for the μ receptor;
- high efficacy;
- rapid metabolism — to minimize systemic accumulation and reduce the risk of systemic side-effects.

EPIDURAL OPIOID INFUSIONS

Continuous infusions of shorter-acting opioids such as fentanyl and alfentanil provide prolonged analgesia. Morphine has also been used in infusions for postoperative pain and the use of patient-controlled analgesia systems have also been reported with epidural opioids.

CURRENTLY USED DRUGS

The dose range of drugs administered by this route is shown in Table 17.2.

Table 17.2 Commonly used opioids for bolus epidural administration

Drug	Dose range (mg)
Pethidine	25–100
Morphine	0.1–10
Diamorphine	0.5–10
Fentanyl	0.1–0.2
Methadone	4–6
Buprenorphine	0.06–0.3
Meptazinol	30–90

Adapted from Morgan (1989)

Morphine

Intrathecal administration of morphine is associated with a more rapid onset of action than after epidural use. The duration of action after intrathecal administration is also longer than after epidural administration with analgesia lasting for up to 24 hours. After epidural administration the analgesia produced by morphine lasts for 8–12 hours. Morphine preparations for epidural and spinal use should be preservative free. The usual preparations of morphine found on the ward contain a preservative, sodium metabisulphite, which may be neurotoxic.

Doses: intrathecal 0.5–1 mg
                epidural 2–5 mg

Diamorphine

This drug has a more rapid onset of analgesia when administered epidurally in comparison with morphine. It has also been used intrathecally to provide prolonged analgesia. It is available as a freeze-dried preparation and therefore contains no preservative.

Doses: intrathecal 0.5–1 mg
                epidural 1–5 mg

Fentanyl

This is the safest and most reliable agent currently used but analgesia is of relatively short duration — approximately 2–3 hours. To counter this short duration of action it has been given by continuous infusion into epidural catheters.

Doses: epidural — bolus 100 μg
               — continuous infusion up to 75 μg/h

GUIDELINES FOR THE SAFE USE OF INTRATHECAL AND EPIDURAL OPIOIDS

Currently, epidural morphine and fentanyl are the most commonly used agents. Several workers have addressed the safety aspects of the use of these agents by this route. Guidelines suggested from an acute pain service in the USA are as follows:

- Careful patient selection with modification of opioid doses for patient age and physical status.
- Regular follow up by skilled and knowledgeable physicians.
- Sound education of all nursing personnel regarding the use and risks of intraspinal opioids including instruction in bedside monitoring techniques which ensure early detection of respiratory depression.
- Provision for periodic nursing updates.
- The use of printed protocols and standard orders developed jointly by physicians and nurses to govern the use of intraspinal narcotics including those permitting immediate intervention by nurses, if necessary.
- Provision of a support system within the hospital which is capable of providing immediate airway management and ventilatory support at all times.
- Continuing quality assurance review of all problems.

(Reproduced with permission from Ready, L.B. and Edwards, W.T. (1990). *Anesthesiology*, 72, 213.)

With adherence to these principles for safe administration, intraspinal opioids may be as safe as intramuscular injections on hospital wards.

18

Inhalational techniques and alternative therapies

Probably the earliest form of inhalational analgesia was the smoking of opium, addicts absorbing the inhaled vaporized drug. More recently the inhalational route has been restricted to the use of a 50 per cent nitrous oxide/oxygen mixture known as entonox. Trichloroethylene and methoxyflurane, both anaesthetic vapours, were once used in low inhaled concentrations for analgesia but have now been withdrawn from use — methoxyflurane due to its nephrotoxic effects, and trichloroethylene as it became commercially unviable.

When the inhalational route is used the blood concentration of the agent reaches an equilibrium at a rate dependent upon the alveolar minute ventilation and the solubility of the agent in the blood. Insoluble agents such as nitrous oxide reach analgesic blood concentrations more rapidly than more soluble agents such as methoxyflurane and trichloroethylene. Similarly once inhalation of the agent has been stopped the analgesic effects of the insoluble agents wear off more rapidly.

ENTONOX

Indications for the use of entonox:

- Analgesia during labour
- Analgesia for short procedures — e.g. dressing changes, drain removal

Nitrous oxide is an anaesthetic gas with potent analgesic effects. However, individual variation is wide with some patients showing marked sedation at inspired concentrations of 30–50 per cent. It is commonly used in general anaesthetic techniques but not as the sole anaesthetic agent.

When used as an analgesic agent it is administered premixed as entonox — 50 per cent nitrous oxide in 50 per cent oxygen. It is distributed in cylinders that are coloured blue with white quartered collars. In some hospitals there may be pipeline supplies of entonox to areas such as obstetric units.

It is a valuable and frequently used analgesic agent. Usually it is given through a two-stage valve — the first stage, a valve to reduce the pressure from the cylinder; the second, a patient-demand valve which opens as a result of the negative pressure generated by inspiration, allowing inhalation on demand. When given from a pipeline, only the second stage is needed. A high flow rate must be supplied to match the peak inspiratory flow particularly in women in labour. Little inspiratory effort is required to trigger the valve and produce a high flow rate. The patient may either inhale through a mask or with a mouthpiece.

Nitrous oxide has a rapid onset and offset of analgesia and there-fore finds a major use in situations where the pain is intermittent, exemplified by the painful contractions of labour or for post-operative patients when physiotherapy, removal of drains, or changes of dressings provoke pain of short duration. Typically analgesic effects are seen after approximately five breaths of entonox. Patients should be instructed to inhale the entonox for a short period of time, approximately 30 seconds, before the painful procedure such as the removal of drains is performed. Once the procedure is complete the inhalation can be stopped. The tech-nique thus requires patient co-operation, especially if analgesia needs to be maintained over a longer period of time.

The entonox mask should be held over the face by the patients themselves. This is a safety feature of this method of administra-tion; should the patient become excessively sedated the mask will fall away from the face. The patient will then breathe room air and rapidly awaken.

Contraindications to the use of entonox

1. Nitrous oxide will equilibrate with spaces containing air and replace the nitrogen. This results in an expansion of air spaces, as the nitrous oxide diffuses into these spaces much more

rapidly than the nitrogen diffuses out. This is important in patients with a pneumothorax, when expansion of the pneumothorax may occur and require urgent drainage. Air in other cavities such as the sinuses, middle ear, and also in the gut, may also expand. Patients with intracranial air following trauma will also be at risk of increasing intracranial pressure with expansion of the air space.

2. Sedation can occur with 50 per cent nitrous oxide and care must be taken in patients with depressed levels of consciousness following trauma or in those given potent opioids.

Advantages

● Rapid onset and offset of analgesic effects.
● Useful for short procedures.
● Administration on demand.
● Patient control.
● Minimal cardiovascular depression.

Disadvantages

● Bone marrow depression with prolonged use.
● Short duration of analgesic effects.
● Continuous inhalation requires effort and co-operation.
● Prolonged inhalation will produce drying of secretions and discomfort.
● Bulky nature of the equipment required for entonox inhalation limits patient mobility.

ALTERNATIVE THERAPIES FOR PAIN CONTROL

Transcutaneous nerve stimulation (TENS)

The application of TENS in the management of pain largely stems from the 'gate' theory described in Chapter 2. This theory suggests that if sensory input from large myelinated fibres ($A\beta$) are stimulated, this would close the gate to painful impulses transmitted by small C fibres. Clinical and experimental pain have both been shown to be reduced by electrical stimulation of peripheral nerves. TENS has been used for postoperative pain following thoracotomy, for analgesia after rib fractures, for acute low back pain, and is now widely used to provide analgesia during the first stage of labour.

The equipment consists of a pulse generator, an amplifier, and electrodes. The electrodes should be carefully applied, using electrode gel to reduce the impedance of the skin, to a site over peripheral nerves supplying the painful area. The frequency and intensity of the stimulus can be adjusted to the individual patient's requirements. Patients may control the equipment themselves after suitable training and familiarization with the equipment, enabling maximum benefit to be obtained. Preoperative preparation and explanation in antenatal clinics in preparation for labour may be especially helpful.

The vast majority of randomised controlled studies of TENS in postoperative and labour pain have failed to show any benefit over placebo. It appears to have no adverse effects and is likely to be of help only with the motivated patient who is keen to avoid other methods of analgesia.

Acupuncture

Traditional acupuncture is associated with the Chinese and has been practised for over 2000 years. The theory behind the insertion of needles at specific acupuncture points is that meridian lines were believed to exist in the body and that imbalance in the body would be expressed as pain. Specific sites along these meridians are related to different organs and regions of the body and appropriate points may be stimulated to relieve pain.

Acupuncture points are stimulated by the insertion of small solid needles into the appropriate location. The needle should be inserted deep into the muscle and a characteristic sensation often described as a tingling or numbness is felt by the patient. Modern techniques include electrical stimulation of the acupuncture needle using a pulse generator.

Acupuncture analgesia may partly be explained by the gate theory but it is also known to release endogenous opioid peptides and it can be reversed with the opioid antagonist naloxone.

19

Antiemetic drugs

Nausea and vomiting are frequent and distressing complications after surgery. In some patients they will occur after a minor body-surface operation associated with a brief general anaesthetic without opioids being used. In other patients their frequency, duration, and severity appear to be related to the magnitude of the procedure, type of anaesthesia, and consequent method of analgesia. Nausea and vomiting are particularly common after gastrointestinal surgery, as a result of postoperative gastrointestinal dysfunction. They may also be an unwanted effect of the drugs that are used to control the pain. Some patients are particularly prone to vomiting and suitable reassurance and support may be important in these patients. Vomiting occurs more often in females than males and is more common in the young than in the elderly.

Vomiting is a reflex response which is controlled and co-ordinated by the brain-stem vomiting centre. This receives input from the medullary chemoreceptor trigger zone, the vestibular centres, cerebellar nuclei, and cerebral cortex (Fig. 19.1).

Afferent pathways from the cerebellar and vestibular centres are susceptible to antagonism by centrally acting anticholinergic drugs, which are useful in treating motion sickness. Dopamine is a facilitatory neurotransmitter in the chemoreceptor trigger zone, receptors being principally of the D_2 type. Dopamine antagonist drugs will have antiemetic properties from action at this site. There is also evidence that dopamine may have peripheral effects on gastrointestinal mechanisms concerned with nausea and vomiting.

Before using pharmacological agents to relieve distress, other remediable causes should be sought. Starvation may be a cause of nausea and vomiting and early postoperative fluids may be therapeutic. Gastric distension resulting from ileus or from air

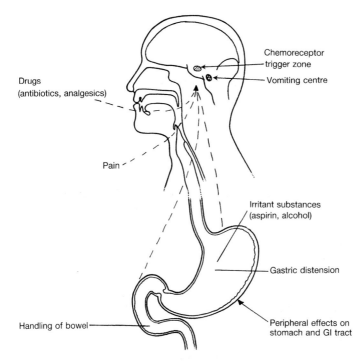

Fig. 19.1 Causes of vomiting and sites of action of antiemetic drugs.

swallowing may cause nausea and vomiting and this can be improved by the insertion of a nasogastric tube for drainage.

Once remediable causes have been excluded, parenteral antiemetic therapy may be necessary to relieve distress. Oral administration may be used for prophylactic antiemetic therapy but once vomiting is established this route is ineffective. Alternatively many antiemetic drugs are available in suppository preparations for rectal administration.

USEFUL ANTIEMETIC DRUGS

Phenothiazine derivatives

These drugs have antiemetic effects which result from their direct actions on the chemoreceptor trigger zone. They are all dopamine antagonists. These agents are the usual drugs for the first-line treatment of opioid-induced nausea and vomiting.

Complications of these drugs include acute dystonia typified by the occulogyric crisis — a distressing combination of involuntary muscular movements and spasm principally involving muscles of the face, head, and neck. This complication should be treated with intravenous procyclidine 5 mg, repeated if necessary after 30 minutes. The reversal of symptoms should occur within 5 minutes of injection.

Extrapyramidal effects are more common in children and the elderly and these drugs should be used with caution in these patient groups.

Chlorpromazine

Administered by injection, orally, or rectally this will reduce vomiting. Complications include hypotension, which results from its α–adrenoceptor blocking action and may be particularly marked in the hypovolaemic patient.

Adult doses: 25–50 mg IM, 3–4 hourly
                    10–25 mg oral, 4–6 hourly
                    100 mg suppository, 6–8 hourly

Prochlorperazine

This drug is used for severe nausea and vomiting and for treatment of symptoms of vertigo and labyrinthine disorders. It is poorly absorbed orally and is usually given parenterally (intravenous or intramuscular).

Adult doses: 12.5 mg IM, 6 hourly
                    5–10 mg oral, 8 hourly (prevention of vomiting)
                    25 mg suppository, 6 hourly

Perphenazine

A useful drug for severe vomiting, this agent is less sedative than chlorpromazine. Extrapyramidal symptoms are more common and the British National Formulary (BNF) suggests it should not be used in children. It too is poorly absorbed orally and must be given parenterally (intravenous or intramuscular).

Adult doses: 5–10 mg IM, 6 hourly (max. 15 mg in 24 h)
                   2–4 mg oral, 8 hourly

Antihistamine drugs

These drugs act on the vomiting centre and vestibular pathways. They tend to be more sedative than other agents. There are no major advantages in antiemetic effect of one antihistamine over another but the drugs do differ markedly in the degree of sedation that occurs with different agents. As a class of drug they are more effective at preventing vomiting associated with motion sickness and middle ear surgery

Cyclizine

In addition to its antihistamine effects this agent also has anticholinergic properties, which can produce unwanted effects of dry mouth and blurring of vision.

Adult doses: 50 mg IV, 8 hourly
                   50 mg IM, 8 hourly
                   50 mg oral, 8 hourly
Children: 1–10 years, 25 mg oral, 8 hourly
                   >10 years, 50 mg IM, 8 hourly

Promethazine

This drug is generally more sedative than cyclizine. It is widely used in obstetric practice or as a premedicant drug.

Adult doses: 25 mg IV
                   25–50 mg IM, 8 hourly
                   25–50 mg oral — daily in divided doses
Children: 1–5 years, 5 mg oral, 8 hourly
                   5–10 years, 10 mg oral, 8 hourly
                   6–12 years, 6.25–12.5 mg IM

Anticholinergic drugs

Antiemetic actions may be peripheral, as a result of antagonism of acetylcholine effects on the gastrointestinal tract and central nervous system effects.

Hyoscine (scopolamine)

This agent is the most widely used, mostly for the protective effect against nausea and vomiting induced by motion and labyrinthine disorders. Its central effects result in pronounced sedation, particularly in the elderly.

Adult doses: 0.2–0.4 mg IM, 8 hourly
                    300 µg oral, 6 hourly

A transdermal preparation is available which releases approximately 500 µg in 72 hours. It should be applied to a hairless area of skin behind the ear. This preparation can decrease the incidence of postoperative nausea and vomiting after out-patient laparoscopy provided it is applied 8–12 hours before induction.

Butyrophenone derivatives

These are centrally acting dopamine antagonist drugs with specific effects upon the chemoreceptor trigger zone. At higher doses, they are major tranquillizing drugs (usually used to control psychotic patients) and have sedative effects. Unwanted extrapyramidal effects are also seen.

Droperidol

This drug is widely used in anaesthesia in combination with opioid drugs for its sedative effects. In low doses it is a good antiemetic following surgery.

Adult doses: 2.5–5 mg IV, 6 hourly
                    2.5–5 mg IM, 6 hourly
                    5 mg oral, 4–8 hourly
Children: 0.5–1 mg daily in divided doses, IM or oral

For vomiting associated with cancer chemotherapy, doses of 20–75 µg/kg IM or IV may be required.

Other dopamine antagonists

Metoclopramide

This drug has central actions closely resembling the phenothiazine antiemetics. In addition, it has peripheral actions upon the gastrointestinal tract. These include an increase in the tone of the lower oesophageal sphincter and increased rate of gastric emptying. The peripheral actions of metoclopramide are antagonized by atropine administration. Extrapyramidal side-effects also occur and are seen most frequently in young female patients.

Adult doses:	5–10 mg IV, 8 hourly
	5–10 mg IM, 6–8 hourly
	10 mg oral, 8 hourly
Children:	<1 year 1 mg, 12 hourly
	1–3 years 1 mg, 8–12 hourly
	3–5 years 2 mg, 8–12 hourly
	5–9 years 2.5 mg, 8–12 hourly
	9–14 years 5 mg, 8–12 hourly

Domperidone

This agent does not readily cross the blood–brain barrier and so is less likely to produce central side-effects such as sedation and acute dystonic reactions. It is an effective antiemetic and is often used in the treatment of nausea and vomiting resulting from cytotoxic chemotherapy. It is no longer available as an intravenous preparation following reports of cardiac arrhythmias associated with administration of the drug by this route.

Adult doses:	10–20 mg oral, 4–8 hourly
	60 mg suppository, 4–8 hourly
Children:	200–400 µg/kg oral

Serotonin antagonists

Ondansetron

This drug was used for antiemesis in patients undergoing chemotherapy and radiotherapy, before being introduced for perioperative antiemesis. It acts by blocking the initiation of vagal vomiting reflex mediated by peripheral $5HT_3$ which is released in the small intestine in response to emetogenic stimuli. It is available as a tablet and for injection. Some studies have suggested that it is better than conventional antiemetics like droperidol especially in established vomiting. Its use is limited by its high cost, usually to a second-line antiemetic and to those with a history of perioperative nausea and vomiting.

For prevention of postoperative nausea and vomiting —

Adult doses: 16mg, 1 h before induction, orally
                    4 mg at induction, IV slowly or IM
Children >2 yrs   100 mcg/kg (max 4 mg), IV slowly

For treatment of postoperative nausea and vomiting —

Adult doses: 4 mg, IM or IV slowly
Children >2 yrs: 100 mcg/kg (max 4 mg), IV slowly

ALTERNATIVE THERAPIES

As drug treatments are only partially effective in preventing or treat-ing postoperative nausea and vomiting, there is greater interest in the use of non pharmacological techniques such as acupuncture, electroacupuncture, TENS, acupoint stimulation, and acupressure. A systematic review of studies using these techniques to prevent postoperative nausea and vomiting found that they were equivalent to antiemetics in preventing vomiting after surgery and were better than placebo in preventing nausea and vomiting within 6 h of surgery. There was no benefit in children with these techniques.

Acupuncture

Traditional Chinese acupuncture techniques have been investigated in the management of postoperative nausea and vomiting and found to be effective. The acupuncture point is known as *Nei-kuan* and is located 5 cm proximal to the most distal wrist crease, between the tendons of palmaris longus and flexor carpi radialis on the right forearm. The needle should be inserted perpendicular to the skin to a depth of approximately 1.5–2.5 cm. Electric stimulation with low current — electro-acupuncture — can be applied to the needle.

Acupressure

This is an alternative where bands maintaining pressure over this position can be worn around the wrist. They have been useful for motion sickness in children but are not effective in postoperative nausea and vomiting.

20
Pain control in special situations

OBSTETRICS

Analgesia for the obstetric patient is unusual in that the doctor must consider two patients — the fetus and the mother — and the effects the chosen method of analgesia will have on both. It is also a situation in which the patient may herself express a preference for particular methods of analgesia.

Analgesia may be required for labour, following operative procedures performed during pregnancy such as cervical cerclage (Shirodkar suture) and after Caesarean section.

Any techniques used during labour should produce efficient relief from pain whilst maintaining consciousness between contractions and good patient co-operation. It should not influence the process of labour. Respiratory depression, particularly of the neonate, should be minimal. Pain relief in labour is a major topic and, other than a brief review, is beyond the scope of this book. Interested readers are referred to the additional reading list for this chapter.

The advantages and disadvantages of the different analgesic techniques in labour are compared in Table 20.1.

Psychological preparation

Psychological and behavioural methods have been widely used in preparation for, and to alleviate the pain of, labour for many centuries. Hypnosis has been used at intervals since it was first described by Mesmer in 1777. Current methods involve relaxation and dissociation techniques, which are taught during pregnancy in preparation for labour.

Table 20.1 The advantages and disadvantages of analgesic techniques during labour

Technique	Advantage	Disadvantage
IM pethidine	Can be given by midwife without prescription. Midwives familiar with effects.	Neonatal respiratory depression. Sedation, nausea, vomiting, and delayed gastric emptying in mother.
PCA opioid (IV)	Allows mother to control analgesic requirements.	As for IM pethidine. PCA pumps are expensive. Training in programming pumps and monitoring mothers needed.
Epidurals	Best mode of analgesia available. Can be continued throughout labour as an infusion. Can be topped up for instrumental or operative deliveries.	Anaesthetist needed for insertion and as standby for problems. Intensive observations needed of mother by midwives. Risk of inadequate analgesia from missed segments or unilateral block. Risk of sometimes rare but serious side-effects including: postdural puncture headache, severe hypotension, local anaesthetic toxicity caused by intravascular migration of catheter, epidural abscess or haematoma causing paraplegia.
TENS	No serious side-effects	Only helpful in well-motivated mother and usually in first stage only. Requires electronic equipment. No convincing evidence of analgesic benefit from studies yet.
Entonox	Rapid onset of analgesia	Rapid offset of analgesia. Euphoria and nausea. Patient co-operation needed. Cylinder/pipeline supply needed.

Sedatives and analgesics

Methods of analgesia have changed over the centuries with the development of potent analgesic and anaesthetic agents. Ether was the first inhalational agent and was introduced in 1847. Analgesia for labour achieved respect following the administration of chloroform 'a la reine' for the birth of Queen Victoria's eighth child in 1853. Inhalational techniques such as entonox (a mixture of nitrous oxide and oxygen) remain popular today.

Combinations of opioid drugs and sedatives — particularly the use of morphine and papaveretum with sedatives such as barbiturates or hyoscine — were common in the first half of the twentieth century. In recent times, pethidine and newer synthetic opioids such as meptazinol have replaced these agents as the standard systemic analgesics.

Regional anaesthetic techniques

Epidural analgesia, whilst providing the opportunity for good analgesia in labour has been associated with increased incidence of instrumental deliveries. Concern over the motor block produced from local anaesthetic agents used in epidural regimes in labour has led to the search for the optimal drug combination, dose, and route of administration. A number of agents have been combined both in infusion-based regimes and intermittent administration either by midwifery staff or by the patient themselves with patient-controlled epidural techniques. These attempts have often been labelled 'mobile' or 'walking' epidurals. The most common combination used in the UK is low doses of fentanyl with lower doses of bupivacaine either by bolus or continuous infusion. Fentanyl doses used are small (30–50 µg bolus, then 10–20 µg per hour by infusion) and there has been no demonstrated opioid effect on the newborn infant.

The advantage of epidural techniques is that they can be rapidly converted to dense anaesthesia, with bolus 'top ups' of bupivacaine, for interventions like forceps deliveries or Caesarean section and for postoperative analgesia.

Episodes of maternal hypoxaemia can occur during normal labour. These are related to cycles of hyperventilation with painful contractions followed by periods of hypoventilation. These can be exacerbated by systemic opioid administration and are generally reduced in nature with epidural analgesia because of the improved pain relief. Epidural opioids in labour do not appear to significantly increase this risk.

Opioid drugs are excreted in breast milk, although the amounts that are present after conventional analgesic regimes are unlikely to produce adverse effects in the neonate.

Transcutaneous nerve stimulation (TENS)

The analgesia provided by continuous painless stimuli applied in the region of a painful stimulus has been interpreted as a 'closing of the gate' to transmission of pain at the spinal cord level (see Chapter 2). For analgesia in labour, external electrical stimulation from two pairs of electrodes attached to either side of the spine in the thoraco-lumbar and sacral regions is used. A low-intensity stimulus is applied continuously with a higher intensity applied during contractions only.

Though TENS is used commonly in the first stage of labour, randomised controlled trials have failed to show any significant effect on labour pain.

CHILDREN

Early research suggested that pain perception and response in infants and children was not established until 3 months of age due to incomplete myelination of pain fibres. Subsequently, clear evidence of cardiorespiratory and hormonal responses to pain has been found showing that neonates do respond to pain.

Variations in sensitivity to pain have not been investigated in older infants and children although it has been suggested that pain thresholds may increase with age. However, younger children will often return to play more quickly after painful procedures and are perceived as having less pain than older children have after equivalent operations. In direct comparison to adults with similarly painful conditions, children receive considerably less analgesia.

Pain control in children is different from adults in the following ways:

- Neonates and premature-infants (i.e. those under 60 weeks postconceptual age) are very sensitive to the respiratory depressant and sedative effects of opioids. Infants should be given opioids only in an area where they can be observed for respiratory depression or excessive sedation and where facilities for ventilatory support is available. Infants who are between three and six months of age may have no greater respiratory depression from opioids than adults although most would prescribe smaller doses of opioid drugs for this age group. Codeine is a suitable weak opioid that can be used in infants on the general ward.
- Assessment of pain in children can be difficult. This is because at different developmental stages, pain is expressed in different ways. In the neonates for example, assessment is usually based on frequency and duration of crying, vital signs, facial expression, and sleeplessness. In older children, from about three years of age, the concept of 'hurt' and that there are varying degrees of it is understood. However, children of this age group find it difficult to express the level of their 'hurt' unless appropriate devices such as picture scales or rungs on a ladder are available to help.
- The intramuscular route, which is a convenient and easy way of giving analgesic drugs to adults, is not popular with children. Children find these injections painful and unpleasant and may become reluctant to ask for analgesia or express their pain.
- Care must be taken over the calculation of doses for children and then in the administration of the correct doses. This may involve several dilutions of the original presentation or the administration of very small volumes of concentrated drug, which can produce errors. Doses may be calculated in terms of body weight or surface area.
- Changes with time: it is important to monitor the effect of analgesics over a period of time to ensure that relief from pain is obtained both initially and during recovery. Other features such as nausea, tiredness, and uncomfortable positions, as

well as psychological factors such as fear and anxiety, can make a child's pain feel worse. These should be noted and managed appropriately.

Aids to the assessment of pain in children

A number of scales for assessing pain in children exist (e.g. CRIES for neonates, OPS for infants and self report scales with visual aides for children older than 3 years). All of the scales use the main principles outlined below in various combinations.

Direct communication

- *Verbalization*: what the child actually says about his/her pain. Self-report scales are the most reliable method of assessment but children must learn how to use them. Listening to the child's description and accepting the level described is important. Criticism of the child and comments such as 'is the pain really that bad?' from adults will make the child agree with the adult.
- *Vocalization*: non-specific crying or whining features.
- *Body language*: pointing to or guarding the painful area.

Indirect, behavioural methods

- *Activity*: a child in pain will be reluctant to move or play.
- *Appearance*: pallor and sweating may be associated with pain.
- *Temperament*: pain is unpleasant and the child may be miserable, withdrawn, and uncooperative. Some children may respond to pain with aggressive behaviour.
- *Interactions with others*: pain may make the child fearful and unresponsive to surroundings or people, preferring to be close to parents with whom they feel secure.

Physiological status

Pain is associated with increased levels of circulating catecholamines. These will produce characteristic physiological changes, which can be used as objective measures of pain. Such monitoring could include the following, which all increase with pain:

- pulse rate
- blood pressure
- respiratory rate

A paediatric pain scoring system is shown in Chapter 2, Fig. 2.3.

Suggestions for improvements in paediatric pain control

Greater use of local anaesthetic techniques

In the intraoperative period local anaesthetic techniques — for example, wound infiltration, caudal epidural blocks, or nerve blocks — could provide postoperative analgesia. These add little extra time to the operation but provide great benefit after recovery from anaesthesia.

Local anaesthetic procedures may be performed during general anaesthesia, then any discomfort which would be felt by an awake child will be avoided. Caudal techniques have been shown to be of benefit for routine surgery such as herniorrhaphy, orchidopexy, and circumcision. These may use either local anaesthetics, such as bupivacaine, on their own or in combination with an opioid. Ilio-inguinal nerve blocks for herniorrhaphy have also been effective. Femoral nerve blocks can be helpful in limb fractures.

More technical procedures such as epidural analgesia are also extremely helpful in major surgery, however the technical expertise and equipment required may mean that these are only available in specialist units.

Continuous intravenous infusions of opioid analgesics

These will reduce the need for unpleasant intramuscular injections and improve postoperative pain relief. The siting of an intravenous cannula can be performed while the child is anaesthetized, when discomfort will be avoided, and venous access may be facilitated by the dilatation of veins produced by volatile anaesthetics such as isoflurane.

It is preferable to maintain a separate intravenous infusion site for the opioid infusion (see Chapters 9 and 10); sequestration of analgesic within intravenous fluids administered through the same cannula can lead to an overdose of analgesic if these other fluids are administered rapidly.

The use of morphine by continuous intravenous infusion to provide good analgesia following major surgery (abdominal and thoracic) in children has been described by Bray (1983). A modified regime is described as:

1. body weight (kg) x 0.5 = milligrams of morphine
2. make up to 50 ml in a syringe pump
3. infusion rate 1–2 ml/h

Patient-controlled analgesia

Children may also use patient-controlled analgesia (see Chapter 10). More recently there has been a trend towards the use of parent- and patient-controlled analgesia or parent-assisted analgesia. In this situation the parent, who is staying in the same room as the child, is also instructed in the use of the PCA system and may, as well as the child, make demands to improve the pain control.

In early reports most parents have found this useful, although others have expressed anxiety about being in charge of the system. No problems have been reported and good analgesia is achieved with this technique.

Use of non-steroidal agents

The relationship of aspirin to paediatric Reye's syndrome may have led to concern over the use of non-steroidal agents. Potential risks of bleeding with their use in postoperative pain may also cause concern. However, they are useful in acute pain regimes and have low incidence of nausea and vomiting. Some NSAIDs can be given systemically, for example, intravenous ketorolac for tonsillectomy, although most are commonly used orally or rectally.

Psychological techniques

Children respond particularly well to psychological interventions (Chapter 4). Treatments that seek to change the level of attention to, or perception of, the pain, including hypnosis and cognitive coping strategies such as distraction and dissociation are also help-

Table 20.2 Guidelines for methods of analgesia by type of operation

Age of child	Minor operation	Intermediate operation	Major operation
<1 yr	Paracetamol	Paracetamol + codeine	Paracetamol + morphine
>1 yr	Paracetamol	Paracetamol + diclofenac + morphine (PCA/NCA)	Paracetamol + diclofenac + morphine (PCA/NCA)

Table 20.3 Doses of analgesic agents

Drug	Dose (mg/kg)	Route	Interval (h)	Preparation (hourly)
Paracetamol	15	PO/PR	4	120 mg/5 ml; 60, 120, 240 mg supps.
Ibuprofen	5	PO	6	Max. 4 doses/day
Codeine phosphate	1	IM/PO/PR (NEVER IV)	8	60 mg/ml or 25 mg/ml syrup
Diclofenac	1	PO/PR	8	12.5, 25, 50, 100 mg supps.
Morphine sulphate	0.1–0.2	IV bolus		As per protocol; see Table 20.4

Reproduced with permission of S. Bass, S. Kinna & R. Sapsford, Addenbrooke's hospital, Cambridge.

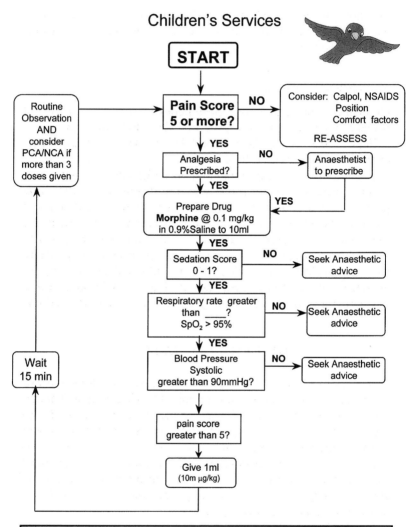

Children's Services

START

Routine Observation AND consider PCA/NCA if more than 3 doses given

Pain Score 5 or more? — NO → Consider: Calpol, NSAIDS / Position / Comfort factors / RE-ASSESS

YES

Analgesia Prescribed? — NO → Anaesthetist to prescribe

YES

Prepare Drug **Morphine** @ 0.1 mg/kg in 0.9%Saline to 10ml ← YES

YES

Sedation Score 0 - 1? — NO → Seek Anaesthetic advice

YES

Respiratory rate greater than ____? SpO$_2$ > 95% — NO → Seek Anaesthetic advice

YES

Blood Pressure Systolic greater than 90mmHg? — NO → Seek Anaesthetic advice

pain score greater than 5?

Give 1ml (10m µg/kg)

Wait 15 min

* <u>Respiratory depression</u>: Draw up 4 µg/Kg of naloxone in 3 mL of 0.9% saline. Give in 1ml increments until respiratory rate is greater than 12 and sedation score less than 2

S. BASS / S.KINNA / R. SAPSFORD. C.N.S ACUTE PAIN MANAGEMENT FEBRUARY 1999.

Fig. 20.1 Guidelines for children receiving intermittent intravenous morphine boluses.

ful. Biofeedback and relaxation techniques may also be useful for painful procedures such as venepuncture in the older child who is afraid of needles.

Management of pain

Guidelines for paediatric postoperative analgesia used at Addenbrooke's Hospital are given in Tables 20.2 and 20.3.

Figure 20.1 shows the protocol for children receiving intermittent intravenous morphine boluses.

The important concept that children suffer pain and that it may require aggressive treatment is only the beginning of improving pain control in children. The differences between children and adults in the expression of pain and the differing requirements for treatment are important. Careful consideration must be given to the child's developmental stage when monitoring the response to pain and analgesia. The wider use of additional techniques, the greater numbers of interested staff available, and future research may hopefully improve the management of acute pain in children.

THE ELDERLY PATIENT

Increasing numbers of elderly patients are presenting for surgery or are admitted with injuries and trauma. The elderly patient shows increased drug sensitivity. Clearance of many drugs is reduced with increasing age because of age-related decreases in both renal and hepatic function. Changes in body weight and lean body mass occur, altering drug distribution. These features explain the need to modify how we administer analgesics in the elderly. *The use of standard analgesic doses in the elderly population may result in the increased incidence of adverse effects.*

Drug pharmacokinetics with delayed clearance should be managed by increasing the time interval between analgesic drug doses to the elderly to prevent drug accumulation. For example, morphine may be administered at six-hourly intervals to a 90-year-old patient, whilst in a fit 18-year-old even three-hourly administration may be insufficient.

Many elderly patients have coexisting medical problems which must be taken into consideration when prescribing analgesia. For example, cardiovascular function may be impaired and congestive cardiac failure may follow from the use of NSAIDs as a result of fluid retention. Elderly patients are also significantly more at risk of renal failure from NSAIDs. In addition, patients with chronic obstructive airways disease may be at increased risk from the respiratory depressant effects of opioid drugs. Epidural administration may be associated with undesirable haemodynamic effects such as marked hypotension in these elderly patients.

Despite these cautions it is important that this group of patients are not deprived of good analgesia. There have been reports of particularly poor provision of analgesia to the elderly and to those who have associated cognitive impairment — a not infrequent complication in the elderly patient with fractures on the orthopaedic wards.

Elderly patients can safely use patient-controlled analgesic regimes with appropriate education and support from nursing staff, with small doses of morphine (1mg), and lock-out times of 5–8 minutes. Continuous infusion techniques should be avoided in older patients because of the risk of drug accumulation.

Increasing awareness of these patients and the combined use of local and regional analgesic techniques after major surgery and trauma should be beneficial in improving pain control in this vulnerable group of patients.

CRITICALLY ILL PATIENTS

It is often difficult to obtain good pain control in these patients whilst avoiding unwanted effects of the drugs. Factors which may contribute to the problems include the following.

- There may be difficulty in assessing pain which may remain unrecognized in a sedated, paralysed patient receiving mechanical ventilation.
- Altered drug sensitivity in the critically ill patient may result in greater adverse effects.
- Reduced hepatic or renal function will delay metabolism and excretion of drugs. Toxic effects may result from the accumulation of the drugs themselves or from the action of metabolites.

- Drug interactions will also be of importance in this group who may be receiving large numbers of drugs during their stay in the intensive care unit.
- Critically ill patients may require treatment for prolonged periods and drug accumulation and side-effects are therefore more likely.
- The respiratory-depressant effects of opioids may hinder weaning of patients from mechanical ventilation, adversely affecting their recovery.

Careful titration of dose and regular assessment of the effect of drugs are essential. Some patients may benefit from the use of regional analgesia. Epidural techniques using opioids or local anaesthetics may be useful for prolonged analgesia in suitable patients. Patient- or nurse-controlled analgesia delivery systems may also be helpful in this group of patients.

21

The acute pain service

DR ANNE COLEMAN, CONSULTANT
ANAESTHETIST, HEXHAM GENERAL
HOSPITAL, NORTHUMBERLAND

For many years acute pain has been managed primarily by junior medical and nursing staff, many of whom have received minimal training to equip them for the task. It is not surprising that numerous studies of hospital patients have shown that acute pain is often poorly controlled, despite many advances in the drugs and techniques available to us.

Management of chronic and terminal pain has developed enormously over the last 25 years, with many patients now receiving psychological, pharmacological, and physical treatments in multidisciplinary pain clinics and hospices. There is now widespread acceptance that these conditions are best managed by staff with specialist training.

Acute pain, however, has not received the same recognition. This may in part be because pain is such a common condition that the expectation is that *all* doctors and nurses should be able to manage it and a specialist approach is therefore unnecessary. The flaw in this argument is that medical and nursing education frequently fails to provide students with the appropriate knowledge and skills.

In the last decade, there has been an increased awareness that acute pain management needs specific training. Acute pain services have been developed to meet this need.

DEVELOPMENT OF ACUTE PAIN SERVICES

The first acute pain service was established in Seattle in 1986 and it was organized in a similar way to chronic pain clinics — patients were referred to the service by their doctors or nurses. A group of specially trained staff (mainly anaesthetists) then took over the responsibility for treating their acute pain. Pain management thus became a recognized specialist activity, for which the patient or the referring physician was charged by the pain service.

This new approach raised awareness of acute pain, but is not easily applied in the largely state-funded health systems of Europe and Australasia. It is expensive to dedicate highly trained physicians exclusively to pain service work and it has the distinct disadvantage that it may further reduce the expertise of junior doctors and nurses in managing pain.

Acute pain services have now become widespread in the UK, but their priorities are a little different from those of the original design in which responsibility for pain treatment was transferred to a team of specialists. **The fundamental role of an acute pain service is now believed to be that of educating ward doctors and nurses to manage acute pain effectively.**

WHAT IS AN ACUTE PAIN SERVICE?

In the UK an acute pain service is a multidisciplinary team which will take responsibility for overseeing pain management in the hospital. In large hospitals there will be staff dedicated solely to acute pain management for at least part of the working week. In smaller hospitals, it is common to combine this role with other duties. The staff of an acute pain service should include an anaesthetist, a nurse specialist, and a pharmacist.

Directors of pain services are usually consultant anaesthetists, as they tend to have the greatest experience of the relevant drugs and techniques and of the management of their potential complications.

Day-to-day patient management is usually delegated to a specialist acute pain nurse who provides the important link between the anaesthetist (who is based in the operating theatre for much of the working day) and the ward staff. The pain nurse should carry a pager and be readily available to provide advice or practical assistance on the wards.

In smaller hospitals, the workload may be insufficient to justify appointment of a specialist nurse. In this case it is important that ward staff have an alternative contact for immediate advice with pain problems. Usually, this will be the on-call anaesthetist.

Whatever the structure, 24-hour availability of skilled advice is an essential feature of a pain service.

A pharmacist is a valuable source of advice, to provide drug information and to assist with preparation of intravenous and epidural infusions.

Ward nursing staff are an essential part of the 'team approach' to pain relief. It is usually helpful to identify a senior nurse from each ward to act as a formal link between the pain service and other ward staff.

Junior medical and surgical staff are often in the front line of acute pain management and should view the pain service as a source of education and support which will help them to treat their patients more effectively.

Whilst senior physicians and surgeons have less day-to-day contact with the service, it is important that they recognize its role and have confidence in the methods of pain relief it promotes.

WHICH HOSPITALS HAVE ACUTE PAIN SERVICES?

With the exception of labour pain, postoperative pain is the most common cause of severe pain experienced by hospital patients. Any hospital undertaking in-patient surgery should therefore establish an acute pain service.

FUNCTIONS OF AN ACUTE PAIN SERVICE

- Education of staff and patients in pain management.
- Responsibility for day-to-day management of pain in the hospital.
- Provision of clinical guidelines on analgesic techniques.
- Audit of efficacy and safety of existing techniques.
- Evaluation of new methods of pain relief.

Staff and patient education

Staff education occurs in two ways. First and foremost is the in-service training offered when the pain service reviews patients. This must be backed up by formal tutorials for all ward staff and written information on relevant pharmacology, physiology, and anatomy. A rolling teaching programme is necessary, so that all new staff can receive training early in their employment

Patient education is increasingly important, particularly when patient-controlled techniques are offered. Verbal and written information is appropriate but the most important feature of all is that information should be *consistent*. Conflicting messages from different members of staff are certain to confuse and undermine the patient's confidence. The pain service has an important role in ensuring that all staff are able to give correct advice or, if uncertain, to direct the patient to someone who can.

Day-to-day management

Day-to-day management of pain control usually involves daily review by the pain service of all patients receiving regional analgesic techniques or intravenous opioid analgesia. Efficacy, side-effects, adequacy of monitoring, and readiness for transfer to oral analgesia should be assessed. Patient education is reinforced and adjuvant analgesia prescribed as necessary. This specialist review is beneficial for the individual patient but is also an important teaching opportunity for ward staff and anaesthetic trainees. Most pain services also welcome student nurses and doctors who wish to join their ward rounds.

The majority of patients reviewed by the service will have recently undergone surgery. The analgesic technique will have been explained preoperatively and started postoperatively by the anaesthetist responsible for the patient in the operating theatre, who will then refer the patient to the pain service for regular postoperative review. However, most services are happy to take referral of patients from any trained member of staff. Common causes of poorly controlled non-surgical pain include acute pancreatitis, pleurisy, herpes zoster infection, and trauma. These all produce acute, severe pain which warrants parenteral opioid therapy or temporary neural blockade.

Clinical guidelines

The pain service is responsible for the provision of guidelines on care of patients receiving parenteral opioid or regional analgesia. In addition to specifying drugs, formulations, and typical dose regimes, these should define the standards of monitoring and patient care appropriate to each technique. These guidelines must be relevant to local conditions (ward geography and staffing levels) and the pain service is responsible for ensuring that safe standards of practice are maintained.

Some units require formal accreditation of competence of individual members of staff and of individual wards when using certain analgesic techniques. Whilst formal accreditation is not yet widespread in the UK, all pain services must have the right to insist on further staff training if deficiencies are identified and to withdraw a particular technique if standards of patient care are inadequate.

Written guidelines should be readily available in all ward areas and given to all new ward staff during their induction period.

If a new analgesic technique is to be introduced, the pain service is responsible for training staff and monitoring practice during a trial period. It is often easier to target one particular ward at first, rather than trying to make changes across the entire hospital.

Audit and evaluation

Audit of postoperative pain relief has been a driving force in the establishment of acute pain services. Local audit allows individual units to identify their own problem areas and seek improvement. Nausea associated with patient-controlled opioid analgesia is a common cause for concern and many units have devised treatment strategies based on their own audit findings. Daily patient review by an experienced nurse specialist provides an ideal framework for both audit and clinical research into new drugs and new methods of drug delivery.

WHAT DOES AN ACUTE PAIN SERVICE *NOT* DO?

New members of staff are sometimes a little confused about the limits of the pain service's activity. The common areas of uncertainty are:

- general medical problems, particularly of fluid balance
- drug prescription
- cancer pain and palliative care
- chronic non-malignant pain.

General medical problems

The pain nurse and/or anaesthetist is sometimes the most experienced member of staff to have reviewed a particular patient that day and may be the first to detect postoperative problems. They will discuss these with ward staff and give advice and assistance when appropriate. However, unless the problem is specifically related to the method of analgesia (or lack of it!) subsequent management should be the responsibility of the ward doctors and nurses.

The most common area for confusion is that of hypotension in the patient receiving epidural analgesia. Hypotension secondary to inappropriately high epidural blockade should always be referred to the pain service. However, when the sensory level is appropriate another cause of hypotension should be sought and the patient should be examined by the ward doctor for signs of hypovolaemia, cardiac disturbance, or sepsis. This is not primarily the task of the pain nurse, although her advice should always be sought if there is uncertainty about the influence of the epidural.

Drug prescription

Prescription of drugs by hospital nursing staff is illegal but increasing numbers of nurses are now authorized to *transcribe* drug orders. Transcription is a process whereby a doctor takes responsibility for a named nurse to authorize delivery of specified drugs to a closely defined patient group. In the pain service, transcription protocols usually concern antiemetic drugs and oral analgesics. At present such protocols are agreed locally and require the approval of the medical director and the hospital pharmacy. If no such transcription protocol exists, the pain nurse must rely on medical staff to prescibe for each individual patient. Conversely, if such an agreement is in place, the pain nurse cannot authorize administration of any drugs *other* than the limited range specified in the protocol.

Cancer pain

Cancer pain can be both severe and acute, in which case the pain service has much to offer in the short term. However, patients with terminal disease require continuing holistic care after the acute episode of pain is controlled, and the relatively invasive parenteral analgesic regimes which dominate the workload of an acute pain service are often inappropriate. Early referral to the local palliative care team is the best course.

Chronic pain

Chronic non-malignant pain is often difficult to manage and does not usually warrant the regional and opioid techniques which are appropriate for acute pain. Successful management relies more on psychological therapy and the acute pain service rarely has the time or resources to deal with these patients adequately. Referral to a chronic pain clinic is recommended.

ADVANTAGES OF AN ACUTE PAIN SERVICE

1. Introduction of an acute pain service has been shown to improve pain relief with both simple and sophisticated techniques. Staff knowledge is improved and incidence of potentially harmful complications is reduced.
2. The development of a structured education programme and readily available advice and help is appreciated by ward nurses and junior medical staff.
3. Optimal analgesia can reduce complications and hence reduce the cost and duration of hospital stay. Some experts believe that an acute pain service can therefore achieve economic savings as well as improving the quality of patient care.
4. The structure of the pain service is ideal for conduct of clinical audit and research.

CONCLUSION

Acute pain services have evolved to address long-standing inadequacies in the treatment of acute pain in our hospitals. They seek to do this by raising awareness of the harmful effects of pain and by educating patients and staff in effective methods of pain control. Whilst specialist skills may be necessary for the initiation of some techniques, the ultimate success of all methods of pain control is dependent upon the ward nursing and medical staff. The acute pain service aims to help *you* to provide effective pain relief.

22

Case studies in pain management

The patient studies in this chapter have been chosen to illustrate commonly encountered problems in the accident and emergency department as well as those in the medical and surgical wards.

Techniques such as regional blockade and the administration of epidural opioids may not be widely available and staff should seek help if unsure about the practice in their particular unit.

In all instances it is important to maintain attention to the patient's general condition and specifically to ensure an adequate airway, oxygenation, and the correction of hypovolaemia or other cause of shock in the individual patient, as necessary.

CASE 1: MAJOR POSTOPERATIVE PAIN

A 53-year-old man has undergone a surgical procedure for repair of a hiatus hernia. The operation was performed through an upper abdominal incision extended into a left thoractomy.

Pain control following procedures such as this can be achieved by a number of methods. The options that may be considered include:

1. Systemic opioids
Acute pain immediately postoperatively is best controlled by intravenous bolus doses of morphine, of 2.5 mg given as often as necessary to control the patient's pain and titrated to the patient's response. An interval of 2–3 minutes should be allowed between doses to allow the morphine to diffuse into the brain and exert its effects.

If available, patient-controlled analgesia systems with intravenous opioids is useful to maintain analgesia, once the pain has been controlled by bolus doses of intravenous morphine. If a PCA system is to be used the patient should be given a full explanation, preoperatively, on how to operate it. The patient should be reassured about the safety of the pump preventing overdosage and how control of analgesia is directly in his or her hands. A full assessment of the patient's ability to use the pump should include their level of understanding and whether there is adequate function in their hands to activate the pump.

2. Epidural anaglesia

This route, using local anaesthetic agents or opioids, is gaining increasing favour as the method of choice for analgesia in these patients. The insertion of catheters into the epidural space is most often performed immediately before the operation by the anaesthetist. It offers intraoperative analgesia as well as continuing analgesia during the early postoperative period.

Useful analgesia has been obtained with morphine and fentanyl alone or in combination with local anaesthetic agents. Local anaesthetic agents, however, are likely to produce sympathetic blockade, which may potentiate hypotension in the hypovolaemic patient. Epidural analgesia may be provided by continuous infusions via the epidural catheter or repeated bolus doses may be given.

For upper abdominal surgery the catheter should be sited in the lower thoracic region. A bolus dose of 5 ml of 0.5 per cent bupivacaine is administered and the extent of analgesia can be checked by loss of sensation to pinprick over the thoracic dermatomes. Infusions of local anaesthetic agents may be used and an appropriate rate would be 5–10 ml of a mixture 0.25 per cent bupivacaine and 2 µg/ml fentanyl per hour. If infusions are used the extent of the block should be checked regularly. Because of the hazards of local anaesthetic agents administered epidurally (for example, hypotension, local anaesthetic toxicity) the patient must be in a high-dependency unit.

Opioid drugs administered by the epidural route include morphine and fentanyl (see Chapter 17). An appropriate dose would be morphine 2 mg, repeated eight-hourly if necessary.

3. Local anaesthetic techniques

Intercostal nerve blocks

An alternative local anaesthetic technique is the use of intercostal nerve blocks. This avoids the effects of sympathetic blockade, provides good analgesia, but may require multiple injections causing discomfort to the patient. There is a small risk of pneumothorax from the procedure. The first blocks may be performed intraoperatively by the surgeon before chest closure, providing analgesia in the early postoperative period.

Interpleural analgesia

Interpleural injection of local anaesthetic is a recent development. Bupivacaine is the most commonly used local anaesthetic and is administered via a catheter inserted between the parietal and visceral pleura; 20 ml of 0.5 per cent bupivacaine is injected through the catheter and this may be repeated at four- to six-hourly intervals.

CASE 2: MAJOR TRAUMA

A 24-year-old man was admitted to hospital after a road traffic accident. He was the front-seat passenger in a car involved in a head-on collision. On assessment in casualty he has fractured the 6th to 10th ribs on the left, has fractures of his left tibia and left forearm, and is deeply unconscious. He has scalp lacerations and is bleeding from his nose and left ear.

The options for analgesia that may be considered include:

1. Systemic opioids

The undesirable side effects of systemic opioids may present a hazard to the multiply-injured trauma patient. Particular problems may be associated with:

- respiratory depression
- depression of the cough reflex
- depression of conscious level
- hypotension

This patient has a serious head injury. If respiratory depression from opioid administration occurs when breathing spontaneously, then the associated increase in the arterial partial pressure of carbon dioxide will increase cerebral blood flow. This, in turn, may cause a significant increase in intracranial pressure, worsening the head injury.

2. Epidural analgesia

There is no place in this patient for epidural techniques, which may also cause elevation of intracranial pressure or exacerbate any hypotension due to hypovolaemia.

3. Local anaesthetic blocks

Interpleural and intercostal blocks can be useful in a trauma patient who is conscious and has sustained multiple rib injuries. In an unconscious patient who is going to need ventilation these significantly increase the risk of pneumothorax and therefore the risks outweigh the benefits.

In this patient anaesthetic assistance should be urgently sought and intermittent positive-pressure ventilation should be instituted rapidly. This ensures adequate oxygenation and ventilation. Opioids may then be used to facilitate mechanical control of ventilation. Fentanyl, along with an anaesthetic induction agent such as thiopentone or propefol, may be given together with a muscle-relaxant drug to facilitate tracheal intubation. These drugs may then be continued as an infusion until the acute phase of the head injury is resolved. The chest injury in this patient (pulmonary contusion, flail segments, and possible aspiration) may also benefit from mechanical ventilation and the respiratory depressant and antitussive effects of the opioids are then useful.

CASE 3: LIMB FRACTURES

An 18-year-old female is admitted with a fractured shaft of femur after a fall from a horse. She is conscious and has no other injuries and is well resuscitated.

This patient will be subjected to several examinations and may need to be moved and X-rayed many times, all of which increase pain, discomfort, and distress. The provision of good pain relief in the accident and emergency department is important. The options for analgesia that may be considered include:

1. *Immobilization of limb and stabilization of fracture*

It is important to note that early stabilization and immobilization of limb fractures will reduce pain. The severity of pain in the affected limb may be aggravated by spasm in muscle groups around the fracture site.

2. *Systemic opioids*

Initially the pain may be controlled by intravenous bolus doses of morphine 2.5 mg, with further intermittent bolus doses parenterally to maintain analgesia until the fractured femur is stabilized.

3. *Inhaled entonox*

This will provide reasonably good analgesia of rapid onset, particularly useful when moving the patient (for example, on to a bed or stretcher), but will require patient co-operation. It is unsuitable for maintenance of analgesia as the patient will need to continue breathing through the mask.

4. *Local anaesthetic blocks: femoral nerve block*

The most suitable technique to provide analgesia in this patient is a femoral nerve block.

Where staff skilled in regional anaesthetic techniques are not available, alternative analgesia must be provided by the parenteral administration of opioid drugs. Whenever a limb fracture occurs, care should be taken to observe the vascular state of the limb. Ischaemia developing in fractured limbs is normally extremely painful. This pain may be abolished with the analgesia produced from regional blockade.

CASE 4: RIB FRACTURES

A 23-year-old man is admitted to hospital after a fall from scaffolding. He has fractures of his right 5th, 6th, and 7th ribs.

The pain restricts his breathing and he develops progressive pulmonary collapse and consolidation.

Multiple fractured ribs are often associated with other injuries, usually after major trauma, and these must be excluded. The problems from the chest injury result from both the alteration of chest-wall mechanics and from underlying pulmonary contusion caused by the injury. Reduction in the chest-wall compliance after rib fractures leads to an increase in the work of breathing, reduced tidal volumes, impaired gas exchange, and development of atelectasis and pneumonia. Analgesia should therefore restore pulmonary function and avoid respiratory depression.

Options for analgesia include:

1. Intercostal nerve blockade

This should include blockade of the fourth to eighth intercostal nerves; 3 ml of bupivacaine 0.25 per cent with adrenaline (epinephrine) should be injected at each intercostal space. Blocks may need to be performed more posteriorly. The injections may need to be repeated eight-hourly.

2. Epidural local anaesthetics and opioids

The insertion of a thoracic epidural catheter requires the assistance of an anaesthetist and therefore this technique may not always be an available option. Doses of local anaesthetics and opioids administered via the epidural route would be similar to those described for the first patient in this section.

3. Interpleural local anaesthetic administration

If a pneumothorax is present in association with the rib fractures the local anaesthetic may be instilled through the chest drain.

Patient-controlled opioid analgesia

The use of patient-controlled systems to deliver intravenous opioids will be useful if these systems are available.

CASE 5: RENAL COLIC

A 35-year-old man presents with severe right-sided loin pain of sudden onset, radiating to the groin. He gives a history of a previous episode of similar pain associated with a ureteric calculus, which was passed spontaneously.

The stretching of the muscle of the ureter as it contracts around the stone during peristalsis causes ischaemia which results in pain. It is referred through the lower thoracic (T11 and T12) and lumbar (L1) nerves. Hyperalgesia in the cutaneous distribution of these nerves may also be felt.

Options for analgesia include:

1. Systemic opioids

The effects of opioids on smooth muscle, increasing tone and spasm, may be a disadvantage in this patient. Pethidine, 75–100 mg IM, or 25 mg IV repeated as necessary to bring the pain under control, is generally regarded as the opioid of choice. Although it does increase smooth-muscle spasm, this effect is less than that produced by morphine.

2. NSAIDs

As a result of the adverse effects of opioids, parenteral NSAIDs have become the analgesics of choice. A suitable regime with diclofenac is 75 mg IM with a further 75 mg IM after 30 minutes if necessary.

As for the management of all acute pain the requirements of analgesia for this patient include a rapid onset of analgesia and minimal circulatory disturbance. A low incidence of nausea and vomiting is desirable to allow the patient to drink freely, a high fluid input being maintained to prevent further stone formation. In addition, the effects of the analgesic drug used upon the smooth muscle of the ureter is important. Maintenance of ureteric peristalsis will increase the likelihood of the calculus being passed spontaneously.

CASE 6: MYOCARDIAL PAIN

A 58-year-old man is admitted with severe central chest pain radiating to the neck and left arm. He has a history of angina on exertion but this pain came on at rest and has not been relieved by nitrates.

The options for analgesia are:

1. Treat the cause when possible

The classical pain of myocardial ischaemia is central chest pain, retrosternal, radiating to the neck, jaw, and left arm. It may be improved by therapy to enhance myocardial perfusion, such as nitrates to decrease the work of the heart and thrombolytic agents (for example, streptokinase) to lyse any thrombus obstructing blood flow to the myocardium.

2. Systemic opioids

Prolonged pain may be associated with crescendo angina or myocardial infarction. Analgesic agents used in this situation should have minimal cardiovascular-depressant effects. The common opioids used are morphine (5–10 mg) or diamorphine (5 mg) given intravenously. Other suitable opioids are meptazinol (100 mg), nalbuphine (10 mg), and buprenorphine (0.3 mg). The pain associated with myocardial infarction will generally only require one or two doses of parenteral opioid.

CASE 7: BURNS

A 45-year-old woman is admitted following a house fire. She has 15–20 per cent burns, mainly around her arms and upper body. There is no evidence of smoke inhalation or airway burns.

In the early stage following severe burns, pain may be a relatively minor problem. Full thickness and deep partial thickness burns are painless. However, pain control over prolonged periods may be necessary in burned patients and may need flexibility to cover the pain and distress of debridement of wounds and dressing changes.

Systemic opioids

Intravenous opioids such as morphine 2.5–5 mg should be given initially to control the pain. If frequent doses are required (every 30–40 minutes) then an infusion of morphine, starting at 5 mg per hour and adjusting up or down as necessary, may be helpful. PCA systems have been used successfully for parenteral opioid administration. Better pain relief in children with burns is achieved when cognitive and behavioural regimes are used in addition to opioid drugs.

Suggested additional reading

CHAPTERS 1–5

Beecher, H.K. (1956a). Relationship of significance of wound to pain experienced. *Journal of the American Medical Association*, **161**:1609–13.

Beecher, H.K. (1956b). The subjective response and reaction to sensation. *American Journal of Medicine*, **20**:107–13.

Budd, K. (1989). Pain: theory and management. In *Scientific foundations of anaesthesia* (ed. C. Scurr, S. Feldman, and N. Soni). Heinemann Medical, Oxford.

Chapman, C.R. (1989). *Assessment of pain in anaesthesia* (ed. W.S. Nimmo and G. Smith). Blackwell Scientific Publications, Oxford.

Chapman, C.R., Casey, K.L., Dubner, R., Foley, K.M., Gracely, R.H., and Reading, A.E. (1985). Pain measurement: an overview. *Pain*, **2**:1–31.

Dickenson, A.H. (1995). Central acute pain mechanisms. *Annals of Medicine*, **27**:223–7

Dodson, M.E. (ed.) (1985). The management of postoperative pain. *Current topics in anaesthesia, Vol. 8*. Edward Arnold, London.

Duthie, D.J.R. (1989). *The physiology and pharmacology of pain in anaesthesia* (ed. W. S. Nimmo and G. Smith). Blackwell Scientific Publications, Oxford.

Egan, K.J. (1989). Psychological issues in postoperative pain in management of postoperative pain. *Anesthesiology Clinics of North America*, **7**:183–92.

Fernandez, E. (1986). A classification system of cognitive coping strategies for pain. *Pain*, **26**: 141–51.

Kehlet, H. (1989). Surgical stress: the role of pain and analgesia. *British Journal of Anaesthesia*, **63**:189–95.

Kehlet, H. (1997). Multimodal approach to control of postoperative pathophysiology and rehabilitation. *British Journal of Anaesthesia*, **78**:606–17.

Kehlet, H. and Dahl, J.B. (1993). The value of 'multimodal' or 'balanced analgesia' in postoperative pain treatment. *Anesthesia and Analgesia*, **77**:1048–5.6

Lambert, D.G. (1998). Recent advances in opioid pharmacology (editorial). *British Journal of Anaesthesia*, **81**:1–2.

Mann, R.D. (ed.) (1988). *The history of the management of pain — from early principles to present practice.* Parthenon, Carnforth, Lancs.

McQuay, H. and Moore, A. (1998). *An evidenced based resource for pain relief.* Oxford University Press.

Melzack, R. and Wall, P.D. (1965). Pain mechanisms: a new theory. *Science,* **150**:971–9.

Nayman, J. (1979). Measurement and control of postoperative pain. *Annals of the Royal College of Surgeons of England,* **61**:419–26.

Ottoson, D. (1983). *Physiology of the nervous system.* Macmillan, London.

Porter, J. and Jick, H. (1980). Addiction rare in patients treated with narcotics. *New England Journal of Medicine,* **302**:123.

Prithvi, Raj P. (ed.) (1995). Pain mechanisms. In *Pain medicine: a comprehensive review.* Mosby, New York.

Remetz, M.S. and Cabin, H.S. (1988). Analgesic therapy in acute myocardial infarction. *Cardiology Clinics,* **6**:29–36.

Smith, G., Power, I., and Cousins, M.J. (1999). Acute pain — is there scientific evidence on which to base treatment? *British Journal of Anaesthesia,* **82**:817–19.

Spencer, R.T. (1989). Drug therapy for pain relief. In: *Clinical pharmacology and nursing management* (3rd edn) (ed. R.T. Spencer, L.W. Nichols, G.B. Lipkin, H.M. Sabo, and F.M. West). J.B. Lippincott Co., Philadelphia.

Taenzer, P., Melzack, R., and Jeans, M.E. (1986). Influence of psychological factors on postoperative pain, mood and analgesic requirements. *Pain,* **24**:331–42.

Treede, Rolf-Detlef (1995). Peripheral acute pain mechanisms. *Annals of Medicine,* **27**: 213–16.

Wall, P.D. (1980). The role of the substantia gelatinosa as a gate control. In *Pain* (ed. J.J. Bonica). Raven Press, New York.

Wilkie, D.J., Holzemer, W.L., Tesler, M.D. *et al.* (1990). Measuring pain quality: validity and reliability of children's and adolescent's pain language. *Pain,* **41**:151–9.

Zhang, W.Y. and Li Wan Po, A. (1996). Analgesic efficacy of paracetamol and its combination with codeine and caffeine in surgical pain: a meta-analysis. *Journal of Clinical Pharmacy and Therapeutics,* **21**(**4**):261–82.

Zimmerman, M. (1979). Peripheral and central nervous mechanisms of nociception, pain and pain therapy. In *Advances in pain research and therapy* (ed. J.J. Bonica). Raven Press, New York.

CHAPTER 6

Benet, L.Z. and Sheiner, L.B. (1985). Pharmacokinetics: the dynamics of drug absorption, distribution, and elimination. In *The pharmacological basis of therapeutics* (ed. A.G. Gilman, L.S. Goodman, T.W. Rall, and F. Murad). Macmillan, London.

Mather, L.E. (1983). Pharmacokinetic and pharmacodynamic factors influencing the choice, dose and route of administration of opiates for acute pain. *Clinics in Anesthesiology*, 1:17–40.
Pleuvry, B.J. (1993). Opioid receptors and their relevance to anaesthesia. *British Journal of Anaesthesia*, 71:119–26.
Pleuvry, B.J. (1996). Opioid receptors — dervation, classification, location and function (including neuropeptides). In: *International practice of anaesthesia* (ed. C. Prys-Roberts and B.R. Brown Jr). Butterworth Heinemann, Oxford.

CHAPTERS 7 AND 8

Bullingham, R.E.S. (ed.) (1983). Opiate analgesia. *Clinics in Anesthesiology*, 1:1. Saunders, London.
Duthie, D.J.R. and Nimmo, W.S. (1987). Adverse effects of opioid analgesic drugs. *British Journal of Anaesthesia*, 59:61–77.
Freye, E. (1987). *Opioid agonists, antagonists and mixed narcotic analgesics: theoretical background and considerations for practical use.* Springer, Berlin.
Hersch, E.V., Ochs, H., Quinn, P., MacAfee, K., Cooper, S.A., Barasch, A. (1993). Narcotic receptor blockade and its effect on the analgesic response to placebo and ibuprofen after oral surgery. *Oral Surgery, Oral Medicine, Oral Pathology*, 65(5):539–46.
Hug, C.C. (1984). Pharmacokinetics and pharmacodynamics of narcotic analgesics. In *Pharmacokinetics of anaesthesia* (ed. C. Prys-Roberts and C.C. Hug Jr). Blackwell Scientific Publications, Oxford.
Jaffe, J.H. and Martin, W.R. (1985). Opioid analgesics and antagonists. In *The pharmacological basis of therapeutics* (ed. A.G. Gilman, L.S. Goodman, T.W. Rall, and F. Murad). Macmillan, London.
Thompson, J.P. and Rowbotham, D.J. (1996). Remifentanil — an opioid for the 21st century (editorial). *British Journal of Anaesthesia*, 76(3):341–2.

CHAPTER 9

Hull, C.J. (1985). Opioid infusions for the management of post-operative pain. In *Acute pain* (ed. G. Smith and B.G. Covino). Butterworth, London.

CHAPTER 10

Ferrante, F.M., Ostheimer, G.W., and Covino, B.G. (ed.) (1990). *Patient controlled analgesia* (2nd edn). Blackwell Scientific Publications, Oxford.

Harmer, M., Rosen, M., and Vickers, M.D. (ed.) (1985). *Patient controlled analgesia*. Blackwell Scientific Publications, Oxford.

Heath, M.L. and Thomas, V.J. (1993). *Patient controlled analgesia — confidence in postoperative pain control*. Oxford Medical Publications, Oxford University Press.

Lehmann, K.A. (1995). New developments in patient controlled post-operative analgesia. *Annals of Medicine*, **27**:271–82.

Mather, L.E. and Owen, H. (1988). The scientific basis of patient-controlled analgesia. *Anaesthesia and Intensive Care*, **16**:427–37.

Owen, H., Mather, L.E., and Rowley, K. (1988). The development and clinical use of patient-controlled analgesia. *Anaesthesia and Intensive Care*, **16**:437–47.

White, P.F. (1988). Use of patient controlled analgesia for management of acute pain. *Journal of the American Medical Association*, **259**: 243–7.

CHAPTER 11

Cashman, J.N. (1996). The mechanism of action of NSAIDs in analgesia. *Drugs*, **52**, **Supplement 5**:13–23.

Cashman, J. and Mcanulty, G. (1995). Nonsteroidal anti-inflammatory drugs in perisurgical pain management. *Drugs*, **49(1)**: 51–70.

Frolich, J.C. (1997). A classification of NSAIDs according to the relative inhibition of cyclooygenase isoenzymes. *Trends in Pharmacological Sciences*, **18**: 30–4

Labrecque, M., Dostaler, L-P., Rousselle, R., Nguyen, T., and Poirier, S. (1994). Efficacy of nonsteroidal anti-inflammatory drugs in the treatment of acute renal colic: a meta-analysis. *Archives of Internal Medicine*, **154**:1381–7.

Watson, M.C., Brookes, S.T., Kirwan, J.R., and Faulkner, A. (1997). Osteoarthritis: the comparative efficacy of non-aspirin non-steroidal anti-inflammatory drugs for the management of osteoarthritis of the knee: a systematic review. *The Cochrane Library*, **Issue 4**.

CHAPTER 12

Markham, A. and Faulds, D. (1996). Ropivacaine — a review of its pharmacology and therapeutic use in regional anaesthesia. *Drugs*, **52(3)**: 429–49.

McClure, J.H. (1996) Ropivacaine. *British Journal of Anaesthesia*, **76(2)**:300–7.

Scott, D.B., Lee, A., Fagan, D., Bowler, G.M.R., Bloomfield, P., and

Lundh, R. (1989). Acute toxicity of ropivacaine compared with that of bupivacaine. *Anesthesia and Analgesia*, **69**:563–9.

Wolff, A.P., Hasselstrom, L., Kerkkamp, H.E., and Gielen, M.J. (1995). Extradural ropivacaine and bupivacaine in hip surgery. *British Journal of Anaesthesia*, **74(4)**:458–60.

CHAPTERS 13–16

Broadley, S.A., Fuller, G.N. (1997). Lumbar puncture needn't be a headache. *British Medical Journal*, **315**:1324–25.

Burstal, R., Wegener, F., Hayes, C., and Lantrys, G. (1998). Epidural analgesia: prospective audit of 1062 patients. *Anaesthesia Intensive Care*, **26**:165–72.

Cousins, M.J. and Bridenbaugh, P.O. (ed.) (1980). *Neural blockade in clinical anesthesia and management of pain*. J.B. Lippincott Co., Philadelphia.

Dalens, B. (1989). Regional anesthesia in children. *Anesthesia and Analgesia*, **68**:654–72.

De Leon-Casasola, O.A. and Lema, M.J. (1996). Postoperative epidural opioid analgesia: what are the choices? *Anesthesia and Analgesia*, **83**:867–75.

Eriksson, E. (1979). *Illustrated handbook in local anaesthesia* (2nd edn). Lloyd-Luke (Medical Books) Ltd, London.

FDA Public Health Advisory (Dec. 1997). Reports of epidural or spinal hematoma with the concurrent use of low molecular weight heparin and spinal/epidural anesthesia or spinal puncture

Horlocker, T.T. and Heit, J.A. (1997). Low molecular weight heparin: biochemistry, pharmacology, perioperative prophylaxis regimes and guidelines for regional anaesthetic management. *Anesthesia and Analgesia*, **85**:874–85.

Lambert, D.H., Hurley, R.J., Hertwig, L., Datta, S. (1997). Role of needle gauge and tip configuration in the production of lumbar puncture headache. *Regional Anaesthesia*, **22(1)**:66–72.

Liu, S., Carpenter, R.L., and Neal, J.M. (1995). Epidural anesthesia and analgesia, their role in postoperative outcome. *Anesthesiology*, **82**:1474–506.

Reynolds, F. (1987). Adverse effects of local anaesthetics. *British Journal of Anaesthesia*, **59**: 78–95.

Scott, D.B., McClure, J., and Wildsmith, J.A.W. (ed.) (1984). *Regional anaesthesia 1884–1984*, Centennial Meeting of Regional Anaesthesia, Information Consulting Medical, Södertälje, Sweden.

Scott, D.B. (1989). *Techniques of regional anaesthesia*. Appleton and Lange/Mediglobe, and Prentice-Hall, New York.

Stafford-Smith, M. (1996). Impaired homeostasis and regional anaesthesia (refresher course outline). *Canadian Journal of Anaesthesia,* **43(5)**:R129–35.
Wulf, H. (1996). Epidural anaesthesia and spinal haematoma. *Canadian Journal of Anaesthesia,* **43**:1260–71.

CHAPTER 17

Chaney, M.A. (1995). Side effects of intrathecal and epidural opioids. *Canadian Journal of Anaesthesia,* **42(10)**:891–903.
Chrubasik, J., Chrubasic, S., and Martin, E. (1993). The ideal epidural opioid – fact or fantasy ? *European Journal of Anaesthesiology,* **10**:79–100.
Cousins, M.J. and Mather, L.E. (1984). Intrathecal and epidural administration of opioids. *Anesthesiology,* **61**:276–310.
Morgan, M. (1989). The rational use of intrathecal and extradural opioids. *British Journal of Anaesthesia,* **63**:165–88.
Ready, L.B. and Edwards, W.T. (1990). *Anesthesiology,* **72**:213.

CHAPTER 18

Finck, A.D. (1985). Nitrous oxide analgesia. In *Nitrous oxide* (ed. E.I. Eger II). Edward Arnold, London.
McQuay H. and Moore, A. (1998). *An evidenced base resource for pain relief.* Oxford University Press, Oxford.

CHAPTER 19

Gillies, H.C., Rogers, H.J., Spector, R.G., and Trounce, J.R. (1986). *A textbook of clinical pharmacology.* Hodder and Stoughton, London.
Grahame-Smith, D.G. (1986). Vomiting and anti-emetic therapy. In *Topics in gastroenterology, Vol. 14* (ed. D.P. Jewell and A. Ireland). Blackwell Scientific Publications, Oxford.
Laurence, D.R. and Bennett, R.N. (1987). *Clinical pharmacology.* Churchill Livingstone, London.
Lee, A., Done, M.L. (1999). The use of non pharmacologic techniques to prevent postoperative nausea and vomiting. A meta-analysis. *Anesthesia and Analgesia,* **88**:1362–9.

CHAPTER 20

Obstetrics

Crawford, J.S. (1982). *Obstetric analgesia and anaesthesia*. Churchill Livingstone, Edinburgh.

Moir, D.D. and Thorburn, J. (1986). *Obstetric anaesthesia and analgesia* (3rd edn). Baillière Tindall, Eastbourne.

Morgan, B.M. (1987). Analgesia in labour. In *Foundations of obstetric anaesthesia* (ed. B.M. Morgan). Farrand Press, London.

Morton, N.S. (1999). Prevention and control of pain in children. *British Journal of Anaesthesia*, **83**:228–39.

Paediatrics

Berde, C.B. (1989). Pediatric postoperative pain management. *Pediatric Clinics of North America — Acute Pain in Children*, **36**:921–39.

Bray, R.J. (1983). Postoperative analgesia provided by morphine infusion in children. *Anaesthesia*, **38**:1075–8.

Lloyd-Thomas, A.R. (1990). Pain management in paediatric patients. *British Journal of Anaesthesia*, **64**:85–104.

McGrath, P.J. and Craig, K.D. (1989). Developmental and psychological factors in children's pain. *Pediatric Clinics of North America — Acute Pain in Children*, **36**:823–36.

Rice, L.J. (1996). Pain management in children (refresher course outline). *Canadian journal of Anaesthesia*, **43(5)**: R155–8.

Schechter, N.L. (1989). The undertreatment of pain in children: an overview. *Pediatric Clinics of North America — Acute Pain in Children*, **36**:781–94.

Thompson, K.L. and Varni, J.W. (1986). A developmental cognitive-biobehavioural approach to pediatric pain assessment. *Pain*, **25**:283–96.

CHAPTER 21

Coleman, S.A. and Booker-Milburn, J. (1996). Audit of post-operative pain control. Influence of a dedicated acute pain nurse. *Anaesthesia*, **51**:1093–6.

Ready, B., Oden, R., Chadwick, H.S., Benedetti, C., Rooke, G.A., Caplan, R. *et al*. (1988). Development of an anesthesiology-based post-operative pain management service. *Anesthesiology*, **68**:100–6.

The Royal College of Surgeons of England And the College of Anaesthetists. (1990). *Report of a working party on pain after surgery*. London.

Wheatley, R.G., Madej, T.H., Jackson, I.J.B., and Hunter, D. (1991).The first year's experience of an acute pain service. *British Journal of Anaesthesia*, **67**:353–9.

Index